Y0-BZC-082

The AMA Book of
Skin and Hair Care

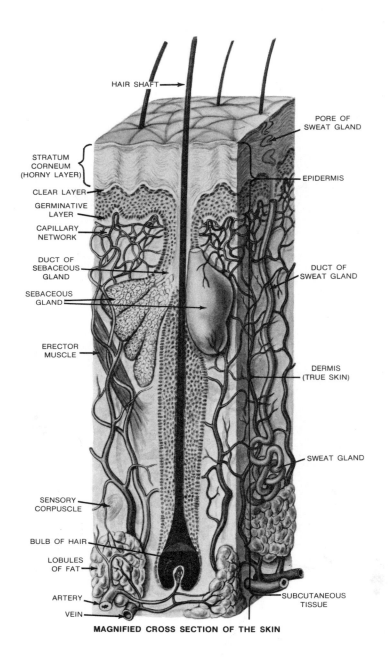

HAIR SHAFT

PORE OF
SWEAT GLAND

STRATUM
CORNEUM
(HORNY LAYER)

EPIDERMIS

CLEAR LAYER

GERMINATIVE
LAYER

CAPILLARY
NETWORK

DUCT OF
SEBACEOUS
GLAND

DUCT OF
SWEAT GLAND

SEBACEOUS
GLAND

ERECTOR
MUSCLE

DERMIS
(TRUE SKIN)

SWEAT GLAND

SENSORY
CORPUSCLE

BULB OF HAIR

LOBULES
OF FAT

ARTERY

VEIN

SUBCUTANEOUS
TISSUE

MAGNIFIED CROSS SECTION OF THE SKIN

The AMA Book of
Skin and Hair Care

Edited by LINDA ALLEN SCHOEN

*Research Associate
Committee on Cutaneous Health and Cosmetics
American Medical Association*

Prepared in Consultation with Members of the
AMA Committee on Cutaneous Health and Cosmetics

Formerly published as *The Look You Like*

J. B. LIPPINCOTT COMPANY
Philadelphia and New York

U.S. Library of Congress Cataloging in Publication Data

Main entry under title:
The AMA book of skin and hair care.
    The 1960 ed., by L. Allen, had title: The
look you like.
    1. Skin—Care and hygiene.   2. Hair—Care and
hygiene.   3. Toilet preparations.   I. Schoen,
Linda Allen.   II. Schoen, Linda Allen. The
look you like.   III. American Medical Association.
Committee on Cutaneous Health and Cosmetics.
RL87.S34   1976   646.7'2   76-7498
ISBN-0-397-01157-1
ISBN-0-397-01158-X (pbk.)

Contents

Foreword

An informed public increasingly interested in personal appearance and skin health demands a basic source of readily available and honest information. Add to this the tremendous proliferation of new cosmetics and cutaneous health-care products, plus new developments in skin surgery, and the need for accurate information becomes apparent. This interest is reflected in the large number of inquiries submitted to the Committee on Cutaneous Health and Cosmetics of the American Medical Association.

All questions received by the Committee have been answered through the years and some were selected for "The Look You Like," a column that for many years appeared as a regular feature of the AMA publication *Today's Health.* Replies were provided by physicians, Ph.D.'s, consultants in the field of cutaneous health and cosmetics, and AMA staff members. We thank the many contributors who gave their time and expertise to provide this information.

Selected questions and answers from the column "The Look You Like" have been published in this book so that a larger number of people will have access to current, authoritative, and unbiased information on the health aspects of cosmetics, common hair and skin problems, and esthetic surgery.

Paul Lazar, M.D.
Chairman
Committee on Cutaneous Health and Cosmetics
American Medical Association

Acknowledgments

The following individuals were members of the AMA Committee on Cutaneous Health and Cosmetics for part or all of the period during which the Committee sponsored "The Look You Like" column in *Today's Health*. Individually they were responsible for many of the answers and collectively for the review of all of the material.

Howard T. Behrman, M.D.
Irvin H. Blank, Ph.D.
Minerva S. Buerk, M.D.
Robert G. Carney, M.D.
Steven Carson, Ph.D.
Marvin E. Chernosky, M.D.
E. Richard Harrell, M.D.
John R. Haserick, M.D.
Harry H. Hays, Ph.D.
Naomi M. Kanof, M.D.
Paul Lazar, M.D.
Arnold J. Lehman, M.D.
Francis W. Lynch, M.D.
Cyril H. March, M.D.
William Montagna, Ph.D.
Carl T. Nelson, M.D.
Rees B. Rees, M.D.
Stephen Rothman, M.D.*
Adolph Rostenberg, Jr., M.D.
Emanuel M. Satulsky, M.D.
John S. Strauss, M.D.
Marion B. Sulzberger, M.D.
Raymond R. Suskind, M.D.

The American Medical Association also expresses its appreciation and gratitude to the following members of its staff in the preparation of this book:

Joseph B. Jerome, Ph.D.: Secretary, Committee on Cutaneous Health and Cosmetics
Valerie Vivian: copy-editor
Laudy Katra, Nancy Lichter, Lorraine Reed, and Iris Scolnick: technical typists

* Deceased.

Part I
COSMETICS

1

Cosmetic Creams

COLD CREAM vs. OTHER CLEANSING CREAMS

Can I use cold cream as an all-purpose cream, or should I use different creams for cleansing, lubricating, and moisturizing?

Cold cream is the prototype of all modern creams—pharmaceutical (medicinal) as well as cosmetic (both cleansing and lubricating). Before the discovery of cold cream about A.D. 150 (supposedly by the great Greek physician Galen) there were only simple salves or unguents.

The original cold cream formula consisted of a mixture of olive oil and beeswax, a maximum of water, and rose petals, added for fragrance. The product was called "cold cream" because when it was applied to the skin the water evaporated, producing a cool feeling.

The oil and wax provided cleansing action by liquefying upon contact with the warm skin to loosen and suspend particles of dirt, oily skin secretions, dead cells, and other material on the skin's surface. They could then be removed easily with a soft cloth. If the cream was left on the skin, it acted as an emollient to soften and smooth the skin and relieve excess dryness.

Cold cream has undergone numerous formulation changes

through centuries of technological and scientific advances. Today the variety of elegant creams, lotions, and foams available show little resemblance to the original, rather simple cold creams. However, the basic formula (oil, wax, water) and the basic purpose (to cleanse and soften the skin) are the starting points of all of these modern products.

Today's basic cold cream is generally a fine, white, glossy cream of firm consistency that spreads with ease and produces a cool feeling. Olive oil has been replaced by mineral oil or combinations of various oils that do not become rancid, as vegetable oils may, and do a better job of cleansing. Beeswax may be replaced by various other waxes and synthetic materials.

Many women still prefer cold cream over other creams, using it for both cleansing and lubricating. Other people find that cold cream is too "heavy" and greasy and prefer one of the modified creams, which are derived from the basic cold cream formula and are discussed in the following answers.

CLEANSING CREAMS

What is the difference between cold cream and the various cleansing creams that are available? Do they have different effects on the skin?

Modern cleansing creams are variations of the basic cold cream formula (oil, wax, water) in which a variety of oils and waxes—plus other ingredients, such as alcohol—may be included. The proportions of oil, wax, and water may be varied, or one of them may be excluded from the formula to change the texture, form, and other physical characteristics of the product or to modify its effects on the skin (for instance, to increase or decrease the cleansing effect).

Generally, cleansing creams are thinner, lighter, have less "drag" on the skin and feel less oily than simple cold creams.

Liquefying cleansing creams consist primarily of oils and

waxes, which melt (liquefy) rapidly upon contact with the skin; they contain little or no water and create a warm rather than cool effect on the skin. Liquefying creams are most often used by women with dry skin.

Creams formulated especially for removing heavy layers of makeup, such as theatrical or masking cosmetics, usually contain a high percentage of oil to facilitate this task.

Cleansing lotions and cleansing aerosol foams are essentially cleansing creams in fluid or foam form. They are often preferred by people who want the feel of liquid with its ease of application; the effects on the skin are essentially the same as those of a cream.

The so-called washable or rinsable creams and lotions are another modification of the basic formula that makes the products water soluble; that is, they may be removed by simply rinsing the face with water (which does not remove regular cream). These products are discussed in more detail later in this chapter.

Creams formulated for dry skin may incorporate ingredients to reduce their oil-removing properties and/or replace oils lost in the cleansing process.

Products formulated for oily skin are modified to remove more of the natural oils and fats from the skin. Of course, people with oily skin may prefer to avoid cleansing creams altogether.

Soap and water are actually more effective than creams for removing certain oily residues and other materials from the skin. On the other hand, makeup—especially waterproof products such as eye makeup or heavy products such as theatrical or masking cosmetics—is more readily removed with cleansing cream than with soap and water.

For many, the most effective skin cleansing procedure consists of using a cream and then washing with soap and water. For others, especially if the skin is excessively dry, alternating the two methods may be preferable. In rare cases of abnormal dryness or in the presence of certain skin diseases, a physician may recommend avoiding the use of soap and water altogether. (See Chapter 16, "Dry Skin, Oily Skin," and Chapter 19, "Soaps and Bathing," for more detailed information on soap vs. cream for cleansing, and on care for different types of skin.)

When cleansing cream (or cold cream) is used to cleanse the skin, it is removed after a few minutes with a soft towel or tissue. A thin film of oil remains on the skin; this can be removed by cleansing with soap and water or with an astringent. If left on the skin, the film will provide limited protection against roughness and dryness. Greater emollient (skin-softening) protection is provided by reapplying a thin layer of cream after cleansing. Emollient creams are discussed in the following answer.

EMOLLIENT CREAMS

The cosmetics counter at the department store in my town seems to be 7 miles long, and every few feet there is a display of different kinds of skin cream—moisturizers, lubricators, night creams, morning creams, ad infinitum. How is the consumer to know which to buy?

Although the many skin products you describe may feel, smell, and look different from one another, basically they are quite similar. They're all variations of the formula for old-fashioned cold cream—but they've been modified so that their primary purpose is to smooth and soften, rather than clean the skin. Because they are to be left on, rather than wiped off, after application, they are made to be less greasy than cold cream.

The majority of these products are mixtures of an oil and water. Other ingredients are often added to prevent spoilage, to keep the oil and water mixed well, and to perfume. Many different kinds of oils, some with very fancy-sounding names, are used—but there is no evidence that one kind is better than another.

If the oil has a low melting point, the oily film on the skin will feel greasy. If the oil has a high melting point, it will not feel greasy; when such a cream is rubbed onto the skin it becomes colorless and seems to vanish; thus the term "vanishing cream." These products are preferred for daytime use and under makeup, when you don't want your face to look or feel greasy.

The purpose of all of these products is to prevent or counteract signs and symptoms of skin dryness. However, it is not possible for externally applied oils—or the skin's natural oils—to keep skin soft and flexible without the aid of water. Indeed, loss of water, not oil, from the outer layer of the skin is the basic cause of dryness. Putting oil on troubled skin will not add moisture to it—and most of the water in the creams evaporates when applied. Very little, if any, is absorbed by the skin.

This is not to say that the products are not valuable. The oily film they leave on the skin retards the evaporation of moisture from the outer layer of skin to help keep it hydrated and flexible. It also makes the skin look and feel soft and smooth by cementing down the rough, scaly surface, and it contributes to smoothness by decreasing the drag felt when touching the skin. There is indeed a wide selection of such products from which to choose. Some women prefer lotions, others oils, drops, or cream. Pick whatever product you like best in terms of feel, fragrance, and, perhaps, your pocketbook. They'll all provide some help.

WASHING CREAMS

How do washing creams differ from regular cleansing creams? Are they a recent development?
So-called washing creams are not really a new development. Formulas for such creams have been available for many years, and a medicated cream making similar claims has been marketed for a long time.

Washing creams are simply variations of regular cleansing

creams. Both contain essentially the same ingredients and have the same cleansing effects. They differ primarily in the method of removal. A cold cream or ordinary cleansing cream is most easily removed from the face with a soft towel or tissue; rinsing with water will not remove the cream or the oily film that remains on the face afterward. Soap and water or an astringent must be used to remove the film. A washing cream is formulated so that it can be completely removed by simply rinsing the face with water. Of course, it can also be removed with a soft towel or tissue, leaving a thin residual film of oil on the skin, if this is desired.

It would appear that the only advantage washing creams offer is easier, faster removal.

COCOA BUTTER AS A CLEANSING CREAM

I have been using cocoa butter as a cleansing cream. Is it of any value? Can it be harmful if used improperly?

Cocoa butter is the solid fat from the roasted seeds of the cacao tree. These seeds are also the source of chocolate and cocoa.

Cocoa butter is an emollient (skin softener) that melts at about body temperature. There is no reason to think it might be harmful. It was once used in many cosmetic creams and in lipsticks, but it is now more widely used in pharmaceutical preparations than in modern cosmetics. It also is a constituent of many suppositories because it softens and melts at a convenient temperature. Cocoa butter alone would probably be more suitable for use as an emollient cream than as a cleansing cream.

PETROLEUM JELLY FOR SKIN

My doctor suggested that I use petroleum jelly on my hands for excessive dryness and irritation, and it has helped. I wonder if it is safe to use petroleum jelly on my face, which also is very dry?

Petroleum jelly (petrolatum) can be safely used on the face to help soften and smooth the skin in the same way as any other emollient. The oily film helps prevent evaporation of moisture from the skin and protects it from irritation. However, petroleum jelly will not go on or come off the skin as readily as a regular cosmetic cream, and it may feel more greasy.

Petroleum jelly, a derivative of petroleum, has been used for a variety of purposes since its introduction more than 100 years ago. It is a common first-aid remedy in family medicine chests as a soothing treatment for minor skin irritations such as scrapes, chafing, and sunburn.

Boys and men who resist fragrant cosmetic hand creams often use petroleum jelly to relieve winter-roughened skin. Many mothers use petroleum jelly to help prevent diaper rash in babies.

Petroleum jelly is included in many cosmetic creams, hand lotions, hair pomades and lotions, lip pomades, and baby products for its emollient effects.

LANOLIN AS A NIGHT CREAM

Would plain lanolin, which is available in drugstores, make a good night cream?

Lanolin alone, like any other semisolid greasy preparation, will help to soften skin and relieve dryness. It is a common ingredient in creams and ointments because it makes such mixtures spread and adhere better to the skin. Lanolin may not be as cosmetically agreeable as a regular cosmetic cream of comparable price because of its tacky smell and because it is difficult to remove. Also, a few people are allergic to lanolin, so it may be advisable to try the product on a small area first.

Various fractions of lanolin have specific qualities, so that fractions or modifications of lanolin are often used in creams and ointments. For example, some fractions are less sensitizing, some are more pleasant cosmetically, and some have better odor qualities.

The most popular form of lanolin for use alone as a cosmetic is hydrous wool fat. For additional information about lanolin in cosmetics, see Chapter 3, "Other Cosmetic Products."

GLYCERIN AND ROSEWATER

I use glycerin and rosewater cream on my face and body but have been told that it is harmful, because the glycerin draws needed moisture out of the skin. I've also heard that glycerin absorbed through the skin can damage internal organs. Is this true?

Glycerin, an important ingredient in many cosmetics, including creams, lotions, deodorants, and lipsticks, is a humectant (a water-attracting agent) and actually helps keep the products moist. It also helps them to spread better. If you applied pure glycerin to your skin, it probably would attract moisture from the skin and dry it out. However, in products such as glycerin and rosewater, the concentration of glycerin is 50 percent or less, and it actually helps retard evaporation of water from the skin.

There is no evidence that glycerin is absorbed through the skin and is harmful to internal organs. In fact, it is often an ingredient in cough drops and some internal medications.

HOW TO APPLY COSMETIC CREAMS

It is sometimes recommended that cosmetic creams and lotions be applied with upward and outward strokes. The reason given is that this lifts the facial muscles upward and thereby prevents sagging of the tissues, particularly in older persons. Does it really make any difference how the product is applied?

The application of cosmetic creams and lotions with upward and outward strokes is of little or no benefit in preventing the natural sagging of tissues that occurs with aging. Sagging of the soft tissues is due to changes including loss of elasticity and stretching of collagen (dermal) fibers, damage from exposure to the sun, and many other factors. With progressive loss of muscle tone, sagging of the muscle tissue also probably occurs to a very slight degree in the aging process.

It is hard to imagine any benefits that could be derived from the technique of "up-stroking." Certainly no such benefits have ever been clearly demonstrated. There may be psychological benefits from this maneuver, as it can make a woman feel she is "doing something."

It is not harmful to apply creams and lotions in this fashion, as long as the application is performed with gentle motions. If the application is performed vigorously, it could stretch or break some elastic fibers of the skin, loosening underlying attachments.

BLEACHING CREAMS

How effective are bleaching creams for lightening freckles and/or other areas of abnormal pigmentation?

There are numerous types of abnormal (excessive) pigmentation of the skin, such as freckles; chloasma, so-called "liver" spots; flat moles; and postinflammatory changes. Bleaches may be of limited benefit in some of these conditions.

The old standard bleaching creams contained ammoniated mercury. Though relatively inefficient, they produced a little lightening of excessive pigmentation. Mercury compounds, however, can cause allergic reactions and other side-effects. For this reason, in 1974 the Federal Food and Drug Administration banned the use of mercury in bleaching creams.

The best lightening agents known today contain hydroquinone. Hydroquinone creams can significantly decrease the amount of pigment; however, these products are useful only for treating limited skin areas where excessive pigmentation results from an abnormal process. They are not useful for lightening normal but "excessively" pigmented skin. In addition, the effectiveness of this chemical may vary between one person and another—and may even vary in different skin areas of the same person. Occasionally, irritation from application of these remedies may increase the amount of pigmentation or may cause complete loss of pigment (leukoderma).

Sometimes, particularly in brown-skinned individuals, inflammatory skin diseases will produce pigment deep in the skin. This usually has a dark black, gray, or blue-black appearance. Since such pigmentation is the result of deeply deposited material, no bleaching product will help.

Increased pigmentation may also result from weathering, primarily from sunlight. In these cases, the skin can be kept lighter if the sun is avoided. Ordinary "suntan" lotions may prevent burning but will not prevent darkening of the skin. To prevent darkening of the skin, a complete sunscreen must be used. See Chapter 20, "Sunlight and the Skin," for more details.

The use of a bleaching cream is a long-term proposition (months or years), during which time the area should not be irritated or exposed to the sun. Melasma (chloasma), also called "the mask of pregnancy," is a type of excessive skin pigmentation common to pregnancy and also fairly common in women taking birth control pills. These unsightly, deeper pigmented areas of the face may require prolonged treatment, sometimes even after discontinuing the pill. See Chapter 15, "Birthmarks—Pigmentation Disorders," for additional information on melasma. Reactions to bleaching creams are discussed in Chapter 4, "Reactions to Cosmetics."

BLEACHING CREAMS FOR REMOVING AGE SPOTS

Is it safe to use skin creams recommended for removing age spots on hands, face and arms?

Preparations promoted for removing age spots and freckles usually contain a chemical called hydroquinone as the active ingredient. It is questionable whether age spots or freckles are significantly lightened by these preparations, even temporarily.

Hydroquinone compounds cause allergic reactions in some people; therefore it is wise to make a patch test to determine sensitivity before using one of these preparations. Apply a small amount of the product to a small area of the skin and check for local irritation or inflammation over a period of 24 to 48 hours. If any type of skin irritation develops, use of bleaching compounds should be discontinued immediately.

For additional information on potential hazards of bleaching creams and the precautions that should be observed when using them, see Chapter 4, "Reactions to Cosmetics." See Chapter 14, "Aging and Wrinkles," for information on age spots.

2

Rejuvenating Cosmetics

HORMONE CREAMS

> *Are the hormone creams marketed by cosmetic firms more beneficial to aging facial skin than conventional emollient creams?*

Most hormone creams available today contain female hormones of the estrogen type. Hormone creams could conceivably act in several ways to counteract many skin changes due to aging.

The epidermis (outer layer of skin) of an elderly person is usually thinner than that of a young person and the surface is drier. Although it has been claimed that locally applied female hormones can cause thickening of the epidermis, there is no evidence that they have this effect on facial skin. Simple emollient creams may help the epidermis retain more water and make the surface smoother, thus relieving the feeling of dryness. These creams also contribute fats to the surface of aging skin, which are sometimes deficient because of decreased oil gland activity, particularly in women. There is no proof that the addition of hormones will make these creams more effective in relieving dryness or in causing an increase in activity of the oil glands.

As age increases, the dermis (supporting fibrous layer of

the skin) also may become thinner and lose some of its capacity to hold water ("plumping"). If the dermis could be made to retain enough water, it would provide better support and would cause wrinkled skin to appear plumper and smoother. The repeated local application of some hormones is claimed by some product manufacturers to promote retention of water in the dermis. Exact measurement of the amount of water held by the dermis is difficult, and there is still no unequivocal proof that locally applied hormones can cause the dermis to retain increased amounts of water.

The fatty layer below the dermis also provides some support for the skin. As a person reaches advanced years, this fatty layer often diminishes—particularly in some areas of the face—with consequent wrinkling and changes in contour. Hormone creams will not restore fat to the subcutaneous layer.

Additional changes related to an "aging look" include degeneration of some components of the dermis (elastic and collagen fibers) from years of exposure to sunlight. Locally applied hormones have been shown *not* to reverse or correct this degeneration.

The federal government permits creams marked to "improve aging skin" to contain relatively low concentrations of female hormones, and cases of overuse sufficient to produce internal effects in adults are rare. However, such products should be kept out of the hands of children.

WATCH THOSE WILD PROMISES

I have seen ads for cosmetic products that claim to erase wrinkles and rejuvenate aging skin so that a person does not need plastic surgery. Are such products really effective?

Man has been looking for the fountain of youth since time immemorial, and the emphasis has never been greater than in today's youth-oriented society. Because aging causes such visible changes in the skin, women and men alike would be happy to delay or reverse these changes. The only problem with products that are marketed to fulfill this desire is that none has ever lived up to its claims.

Assertions are made that products with secret formulas are "available to women over thirty-five who desire to retain or regain a more youthful appearance of the face and neck." The careful reader knows that this is neither a guarantee nor a promise that the product will work. There seems to be a never-ending supply of these products; the only differences among them are in the exotic ingredients that are supposed to supply the benefits.

Today, natural proteins and polyunsaturates are popular as ingredients for exaggerated promotions. Evidently the promoters believe that, since polyunsaturates are receiving so much attention in regard to diet, they can also be promoted for "feeding" aging skin. However, we are aware of no valid scientific evidence to support cosmetic claims for these ingredients.

Equally misleading are those products containing mysterious ingredients such as "Formula X-9," or placenta extract, "milk serum," or aloe vera. The promoters of such preparations use suggestive advertising techniques alluding to flimsily conducted experiments reported under the guise of scientific research. We urge women to exercise the same basic good judgment when purchasing cosmetics that they use when shopping for other goods.

Where applicable, esthetic surgery performed by a qualified physician provides today's most rewarding approach to enhancing the appearance of the skin. Cosmetic products, artfully used, are capable of making minor to marked improvements in appearance by enhancement of natural endowments or masking of what are felt to be defects.

ALGAE IN COSMETICS

There is a cosmetic product on the market that claims to contain algae for fending off lines and wrinkles and for giving skin moisture protection. Is this product safe?

There is no scientific evidence that algae (simple plants such as seaweed and pond scum), when incorporated into cosmetics, provide any special therapeutic or rejuvenating benefits.

The product would not be harmful to use (the concentration of algae is probably low), but it would not be any more helpful than a cream or lotion without any "special" or "exotic" ingredients.

Any emollient cream or lotion will help to soften the skin and retard the evaporation of moisture, thus helping to relieve dry skin.

ALOE VERA COSMETICS

Does aloe vera juice in cosmetics provide special benefits? I understand that aloe vera has been used since ancient times because of its therapeutic qualities.

Several drug and cosmetic products on the market claim to contain "aloe vera" juice, for which special claims are made. There is no scientific evidence that this juice provides any special benefits alone or in such preparations.

Aloe vera juice is the slightly turbid, colored, untreated juice from the aloe plant leaf. It contains 99.5 percent water; the remaining 0.5 percent includes some 20 amino acids and carbohydrates. None of these appears to have the kind of activity that would lend even small support to the therapeutic claims.

There also is some question as to the exact identification of the source plants for the juice. Aloe vera is frequently advertised as a "drug of the Bible." The aloe mentioned in ancient literature refers to a substance that was used as a spice or an incense, and therefore was quite different from the modern commercial juice. Aloe vera juice also has little in common with the drug aloe, which is a laxative.

Claims for therapeutic effects of aloe vera depend primarily on testimonials rather than on reports of well-controlled, objective studies.

MINK OIL OND TURTLE OIL COSMETICS

What special benefits do exotic ingredients such as mink oil and turtle oil provide when added to cosmetic preparations?

Various exotic ingredients incorporated into cosmetic preparations have been touted over the years as providing special benefits for the skin. There are no scientific data to support such claims.

A few years ago, it seemed that mink oil and turtle oil had finally passed into history as cosmetic ingredients. But recently products with these ingredients have again been marketed. It is generally agreed that application of oil to the skin helps relieve dryness and temporarily improves the appearance of fine lines and wrinkles, because oil helps to minimize evaporation of moisture from the skin. By smoothing the surface scales of excessively dry skin, oil helps to make the skin look and feel softer.

However, there is no published scientific proof for claims that turtle oil or mink oil are superior to the oils commonly used in cosmetic preparations. The only apparent reason for inclusion of these and most other exotic ingredients in cosmetic preparations is that they make good advertising copy.

Since mink coats are expensive and beautiful, cosmetics containing mink oils are supposed to be "beautiful" and help make the wearer "beautiful." Aside from the fact that turtles are known to live long, we can't imagine why turtle oil is considered a desirable cosmetic ingredient. Actually, a turtle has very unattractive skin by the prevalent standards of feminine beauty.

Such cosmetic products depend for their appeal on human vanity and the desire to be young and beautiful. Unfortunately, no cosmetic preparation—whether it contains turtle oil, mink oil, royal jelly, or any other exotic or "secret" ingredient—will provide youth and beauty.

The realistic person will accept the limitations of cosmetics as well as their benefits. Cosmetics *cannot* perform miracles. They *can* add color to the skin and hair, help conceal minor blemishes, and temporarily relieve excessive skin dryness or oiliness. In this way cosmetics help people to look and feel more attractive. But they accomplish this solely through their basic properties such as color, fragrance, and local physical action.

COLLAGEN COSMETICS

Recently I've seen a lot of advertisements for cosmetics with collagen. What is collagen? Does it do anything special for the skin?

Collagen may be the current "wonder" ingredient in the cosmetic world's coffers—but it doesn't appear to do much for the skin. Advertisements implying anything to the contrary are misleading.

Collagen is a protein substance found in the connective tissue, cartilage, and bone of the body. While changes in collagen fibers contribute to wrinkles and the appearance of aging skin, adding collagen to any cosmetic will not affect collagen in the skin or in any way reverse the changes that have taken place. There is no evidence that collagen in the skin can be affected by any cosmetic—whether or not it contains collagen. You won't look any younger as a result of using collagen cosmetics.

3

Other Cosmetic Products

MATTE-FINISH MAKEUP

> *How do matte-finish, all-in-one makeups differ from regular liquid makeup bases? Are they more drying or more harmful to the skin than ordinary makeups?*

Matte-finish cream makeups are essentially more concentrated versions of standard makeups. They are designed to simulate the effect of a liquid makeup plus a light covering of face powder. This means that matte-finish products must contain more powder and pigment. Hence, they produce less sheen on normal skin than standard, tinted, liquid makeups.

Since these products also contain more emollient materials, they probably are no more drying to the skin than standard liquid makeups.

FROSTED MAKEUP

> *Brush-on makeup powders that seem to contain tiny bits of metal to give a frosted look or glitter finish are being sold. What is this metal? Are the powders harmful?*

Frosted or "pearlized" makeup has become popular in recent years, particularly in the pressed-powder, brush-on forms. Frosted lipsticks and nail polishes have been available for some time.

Guanine, a natural pearl substance obtained from the scales of certain fish, was used originally as the sparkle material in most makeup preparations. Today, most manufacturers use either synthetic pearl (bismuth oxychloride) or aluminum and bronze particles. The manufacturing process of aluminum and bronze particles for use in cosmetics is highly controlled; the particles produced are of a special size and have rounded edges to minimize abrasiveness. In addition, a transparent coating is often applied to these particles.

Guanine and bismuth oxychloride are considered nontoxic and harmless for use in cosmetics; the aluminum and bronze pigments are considered generally safe for use except in the eye area. Of course, some people develop an allergic reaction to this type of makeup much the same as to other cosmetics. There are also specially formulated cosmetics for sensitive skins that are available in frosted forms.

TRANSLUCENT POWDER

What is the difference between translucent and "ordinary" face powder? I've heard that the translucent kind contains silicone particles and should be kept away from the eyes.

The only difference between translucent and "ordinary" face powder is the degree of opacity. Translucent makeups are, surprisingly, more opaque. This effect is achieved by titanium dioxide, a standard material long used in makeup.

Face powders and makeups contain silicates, commonly known as talcs. Talcs come in many qualities and degrees of fineness. The quality used in cosmetics is extremely good, and any particle that might accidentally become dusted into the eye during use would cause no damage.

Silica, also called silicon dioxide, occurs in nature in several forms including sand, rock crystal, and quartz. However, these are not used in makeup because of their excessive hardness. (Many silicates, on the other hand, are remarkably soft.)

Silicones are polymerized substances quite different from both silicates and silica. In the cosmetics and makeup industry, the best known silicone is dimethyl polysiloxane. Reports that cosmetics containing silicones, such as some hand lotions, may cause redness and irritation of the eyelids upon accidental contact are not supported by clinical evidence.

UNDERMAKEUP COLOR TONERS

My face has a tendency to be red and flushed and therefore unattractive. My physician says there is nothing wrong with me. I have tried all kinds of regular makeups, but none seems to help. If I put on enough to conceal the redness, I look heavily made up. Can you suggest anything that might help me?

If your physician can find no underlying medical problem to explain the red, flushing appearance, it is probable that you simply have a ruddy complexion. If this is the case, it cannot be permanently altered. However, overexposure to the sun and factors that cause flushing—such as steam baths, saunas, hot foods, and alcohol—should be avoided, since they may exaggerate the redness.

Cosmetics offer the most practical solution for concealing redness. If regular cosmetics have proved ineffective, you may want to try one of the undermakeup toners that several cosmetic firms offer. Applied as a film under regular makeup, they help to even out skin-color tones such as red blotches or irregular patches of color. They can also help brighten sallow-toned complexions or give a tanned look to the skin, depending on the shade used. The film produces a color effect that resembles staining; this color is removed by soap and water or cleansing cream.

Undermakeup toners are available in several forms—liquids, creams, gels, and sticks—and in various colors. For example, green colors are intended to tone down florid (red) complexions, browns give a tanned look to the skin. If toners are not adequate for evening out the color of your complexion, you may want to try special masking cosmetics, which are designed primarily to cover birthmarks. Some popular brands of cosmetics also include a masking foundation in their lines.

You may want to consult a cosmetician about under-makeup toners and masking cosmetics for your particular complexion.

MAKEUP FOR MASKING BIRTHMARKS

Is there any special type of cosmetic I can use to cover a birthmark? Regular makeup is ineffective.
Many types of cosmetics are available to cover unsightly marks. Most of these preparations are creams containing masking agents such as titanium dioxide and zinc oxide. Pigments are added to give a range of colors. Various lipsticklike applicators or sticks that contain similar color bases are also available. These are often effective for masking small areas.

You would probably achieve greater satisfaction by consulting a dermatologist, who can recommend either a specific type of product or a formulation that has been found of value. A dermatologist can also tell you about treatments by which certain types of birthmarks can be removed or made less noticeable. "Covermark" is one brand of products specifically designed for masking cosmetic defects due to birthmarks.

SKIN FRESHENERS AND ASTRINGENTS

What are skin fresheners and astringents, and when should they be used?
Fresheners are clear liquids made of alcohol, water, and glycerin. The alcohol makes the skin feel cool and refreshed, and these preparations are useful for quick removal of makeup and between-time cleansing.

Astringents have a higher concentration of alcohol than

fresheners and may contain additional ingredients such as boric acid, alum, menthol, and camphor. In addition to making the skin feel refreshed, they give it a tightened feeling. There is no evidence that pores can be shrunk by the use of these preparations. Overuse should be avoided by persons with dry skin.

Although astringents are usually promoted for oily skin, both fresheners and astringents may be used effectively for other types of skin as well.

MEDICATED COSMETICS

Are medicated cosmetics better than others?
The practice of incorporating antibacterial agents into soaps, cosmetics, and other toilet preparations has increased markedly in recent years. Makeup, lipstick, shaving cream, shampoo, toilet soap, and many other regularly used preparations are now available in "medicated" form. The names of the active ingredients usually appear on the product labels.

While these agents are useful in medical preparations for the treatment of minor cuts and abrasions, in cosmetics and toilet preparations they work primarily to limit bacterial contamination of the *product* (not the user) during the period of use.

Furthermore, their potential harm often outweighs their benefits. People can become allergic to these antibacterial ingredients, and thereby allergic to many other commonly used products that contain the same ingredients. Physicians have reported that those who become sensitive to certain anti-infective agents may also exhibit a sensitivity to chemically related compounds. Since these agents appear in a growing number of commonly used preparations, the possibility of such cross-sensitization is increasing greatly. Some of these agents are also known to cause contact photodermatitis (skin reactions caused by the action of sunlight or other strong light). Medicated cosmetics should not be confused with the so-called hypoallergenic cosmetics that are discussed in Chapter 5, "Cosmetics—Miscellaneous."

FRAGRANCE FORMULATIONS

How do perfume, cologne, and toilet water differ?
Perfume is created from a chemical formulation of fragrant volatile oils, preservatives, and alcohol. The oils are obtained from a variety of sources, including spices, flowers, and fruits. Perfume has a stronger fragrance than cologne or toilet water.

Toilet water is made by using large amounts of alcohol in the perfume formula. The scent is similar to that of perfume but does not last as long and is not as strong.

Cologne is similar to toilet water, and the terms are often used synonymously. However, cologne is generally limited to citrus and floral bases.

Cologne and toilet water are usually applied more liberally than perfume. The fragrances are lighter, and the higher alcohol content gives a cooling, refreshing feel to the skin.

WHITE LIPSTICK

Is there any possibility of harm resulting from the use of white lipstick?
White lipstick is nothing more than ordinary lipstick in which the dyes or colored pigments have been replaced by a white pigment, ordinarily titanium dioxide. In addition to the white pigment, it may contain bismuth oxychloride or guanine to give a "pearlized" effect. These ingredients are generally considered safe for use in cosmetics.

LIPSTICK COLOR CHANGES

Every lipstick I buy changes color while I'm wearing it. A bluish-red color develops. The salespeople tell me it's because I have too much acid in my system. Is this true?

Is there any way to correct the problem or are there any lipsticks that won't change color?

Lipsticks do not really change color. The color will often appear different in different lighting, especially fluorescent lighting, but this is not a true color change. A few women observe a bluish-red color at varying periods of time after application. Actually, this means it's time to reapply the lipstick because its real color has worn off.

Lipstick consists of two color components. The first provides the "true" color—the color you see as you observe the lipstick in its case or the line it will make as you stroke it on your skin. The other component provides the adhering or staying power of the lipstick to the natural vermilion of your lips. This portion does not rub off with ordinary wear because it has become an intimate part of your skin surface. Regardless of the shade of lipstick you select, the basic color of the second component always has a bluish tinge. The bluish coloration occasionally noted really means that the true color component of the lipstick has worn off and the second, adhering component remains. Obviously, reapplication will correct the color change.

It is possible to reduce the tendency for this color alteration by selecting lipsticks in the yellow family of colors. The tendency to change color will also be reduced if the lipstick is applied to lips that have been freshly cleansed.

MASCARA

What are the differences among the various kinds of mascara? Can they harm the eyelashes?

Mascara is generally a combination of soap, wax, or liquid along with color pigments designed to color the eyelashes. It's all basically the same. Cake mascara made with a wax formula is first wet with water, then applied with a brush. It is moderately water resistant. Cream mascara, an aqueous emulsion, comes in a tube and is applied with a brush. Liquid mascara is similar to the cream type, but generally comes in an automatic pencil-like container with a built-in brush-type applicator. It's also more water resistant than cake mascara.

The new "lash-extender" mascara is really liquid mascara with tiny synthetic fibers added. As the liquid evaporates, the fibers adhere to the wet lashes, making them appear thicker and longer.

Modern mascara preparations generally do not damage the eyelashes or eye area. Only safe, insoluble color pigments (not dyes) are permitted in eye makeup.

Mascara rarely produces allergic reactions. However, to guard against possible infections, no eye makeup should ever be loaned or borrowed.

WATERPROOF EYELINER

I have a waterproof eyeliner that came with a remover. If a remover is necessary, I wonder whether the product is safe to use.

There are two categories of waterproof cosmetics: (1) those that resist tears, moisture in the air, and perspiration; and (2) those that resist all three of these plus ordinary soap and water. The second type requires some other means of removal. This is no reflection on the safety of the product.

Makeup products that are resistant to soap and water generally can be removed with a solvent such as mineral oil or similar oils. Most facial cleansing creams, oils, and lotions, as well as most eye-makeup removers, contain one or more of these solvents as basic ingredients, so any of these products may effectively remove waterproof eye makeup.

All makeup products should be removed before retiring to avoid skin problems that can arise from wearing excessive or oily cosmetics over extended periods of time. Where makeup is not readily removed by soap and water, a special remover may be easier to use.

It is doubtful that any eye makeup is completely waterproof. However, products advertised as waterproof generally remain in place longer than products that do not make this claim.

Many waterproof eye cosmetics are, in the simplest terms, composed of either a pigmented waxy base dissolved in a volatile solvent or a pigment suspended in a gum or resin solution. The latter are responsible for eyeliners that dry to a glossy finish and take on the plasticlike consistency that allows them simply to be "peeled" off. (See the following exchange for information on the safety of eye cosmetics.)

EYE-COSMETIC SAFETY

How safe are eye cosmetics?
Regulations govern all cosmetics to be used around the eyes. Ingredients that may damage the eyes—certain dyes and colors —may not be used.

Because eyelids are easily irritated, eye makeup, particularly eyeliner, should be removed with care. Too frequent or harsh cleansing may cause irritation to the lid surface. Eye makeup should not be removed and reapplied repeatedly at one session. If you are not satisfied with the initial application, it is advisable either to make do or to remove the eye makeup completely and wait a few hours before reapplying it.

The thin skin of the eyelids is particularly susceptible to contact dermatitis (inflammation of the skin) from various causes, particularly cosmetics. Allergic reactions near the eyes often are caused by cosmetic preparations designed for use on other body areas—especially hair preparations and nail polish. However, some people are allergic to eye makeup. If your skin becomes red, itchy, or swollen whenever an eye cosmetic is applied, you may be allergic to one or more ingredients in the product—and you should stop using it.

Sometimes an allergy is caused by ingredients used in only one brand of cosmetics, and changing brands will solve the problem. Some products do not contain the ingredients most often responsible for allergic reactions. In a few cases, the use of eye makeup must be stopped altogether. If the reaction is severe, persistent, or recurrent, see a physician for treatment.

MERCURY IN COSMETICS

My mother tells me that there's mercury in cosmetics, especially eye shadow. Does this pose a danger to my health?

The Federal Food and Drug Administration has banned the use of mercury compounds in all cosmetics except eye makeup.

Very small concentrations of mercury (less than 0.1 percent) in the form of phenyl mercuric salts are used in eye cosmetics as a preservative to inhibit the growth of microorganisms. There is no evidence at present that mercury from these products is absorbed through the skin into the body in harmful amounts.

In eye cosmetics, where no satisfactory substitute preservative exists, the risk of using the mercury compound is considered much less than the risk of using no preservatives. One "built-in" safety factor is that cosmetic eye preparations are used in small amounts and applied to limited areas of the body.

COSMETICS AND CONTACT LENSES

I recently started wearing contact lenses. Should I take any special precautions in regard to wearing cosmetics?

Cosmetics can present problems for a wearer of contact lenses if they get on the lens or into the eye. Many problems can be eliminated if you follow these precautions:

- Apply cosmetics after inserting lenses.
- Avoid using an oily agent when lenses are being worn. It will adhere to the lenses and cause blurring of vision.

- Use cosmetics sparingly around the eyelids.
- Use only waterproof mascara. Do not use "lash-extender" mascara, because this contains tiny fibers that may enter the eye, become trapped under the lens and cause discomfort.
- When hair spray is used, keep your eyes closed during application and for a few minutes afterward to allow the mist to settle out of the air.
- Do not use hand cream or lotion before inserting contacts; they will produce an oily film that may cloud the lenses.

Cosmetics can be removed from lenses by washing them with a commercial contact lens cleansing solution. If irritation develops, stop wearing the lenses and see your ophthalmologist.

FALSE EYELASHES AND CONTACT LENSES

Can a person who wears contact lenses safely wear false eyelashes? Is it harmful if eyelash adhesive gets into the eyes or on the lenses?

It is safe to wear regular false eyelashes and contact lenses. (See the following exchange for a discussion of semipermanent false lashes.)

The glue used for the eyelashes, if allowed to come in contact with the lens, does not permanently damage the lens. It can be removed by many of the lens cleaners now available.

Eyelash adhesive, as any foreign substance, can cause discomfort if it gets into the eyes. If irritation is excessive, wearing the lenses should be postponed until the patient's physician advises resumption of their use.

SEMIPERMANENT FALSE EYELASHES

A friend keeps trying to convince me to invest in the semipermanent false eyelashes available at beauty salons.

*These lashes are applied individually and are supposed to
look very natural. But I wonder how good they really are.*
Semipermanent false eyelashes are expensive, probably will not
last as long as implied, and can cause trouble medically. If
hypoallergenic surgical adhesive is used to attach the lashes
(they're glued, individually, to your own eyelashes, eliminating
the eyelid band), there shouldn't be any problem. Sometimes,
however, epoxy glue is used because of its greater holding
power—and epoxy glue is too strong and dangerous to be used
in the eye area. It can easily get onto your eyelid and even into
your eye.

As the false lashes become unglued—they shouldn't be
expected to last more than two or three weeks, if that long—
they might fall into your eye. Since the false lashes may be
longer or stiffer than your natural lashes, they'll be even more
irritating. And the missing lashes have to be replaced—at additional cost.

Semipermanent lashes are definitely not recommended for
contact-lens wearers (they'll have to settle for the regular
band-type false eyelashes if they want to go this route). A
fallen eyelash lodged beneath a contact lens can produce
severe irritation or even corneal abrasion. Epoxy glue, if used,
can get on the lens and damage the surface.

If you try the new lashes and incur any eye irritation,
check with an ophthalmologist.

LEMON AIDS

*Many cosmetic companies boast that their products con-
tain lemon. What good does lemon do for skin and hair?*
Not as much good as some ads lead you to believe. Lemon
juice is a mild acid. When used as a rinse after shampooing
in hard water with soap shampoo, it rinses away soap scum and
makes hair look brighter and shinier.

Today, however, most shampoos are made with synthetic

detergents instead of soap. These don't cause soap scum to stick to hair, so a lemon rinse is not needed.

In fact, most products that claim to contain lemon actually contain a lemon extract with almost no acidic content at all. These products give off a pleasant but short-lived lemony fragrance, which is about all the lemon ingredient accomplishes. We know of no scientific evidence to support manufacturers' claims that lemon juice enhances the value of skin creams, acne preparations, lotions, etc. Indeed, lemon juice or oils from lemon peel in such products can produce allergic reactions in people with sensitive skin. It appears to us that lemon extracts are added to cosmetic products primarily for their advertising value.

EGG FACIALS

I've tried many different homemade facials, but haven't been satisfied. Now I've heard about the egg treatment. How much of the egg do you use and how do you use it? You may not be any more satisfied with an egg facial than with others you have tried if you're expecting a great change in your skin. The effects of facials, egg or otherwise, are primarily psychological.

As the facial dries, it tightens and pulls the skin, making the user think something must be happening. When the facial is rinsed off, surface skin debris is removed along with the facial mask and the skin feels cleaner and refreshed. For the most part facials are not harmful, although people with exceptionally dry skin may find them irritating.

If you want to try an egg facial, use only the white or albumin. Beat the whites until they are light and fluffy, as for meringues, then apply them to your face and neck, allow them to dry, and remove the masque with cold water.

ORGANIC COSMETICS

What is your opinion of the organic cosmetics that are now popular? Are they better for the skin than cosmetics with chemical ingredients?

There is little or no scientific basis for the claim that organic cosmetic ingredients (extracts from fruits, vegetables, herbs, or other plants) provide special benefits to skin. Originally, cosmetics were made from these ingredients because nothing else was available. They have since been replaced by synthetic ingredients because the latter provide a wider range of colors, last longer on the skin, cleanse better, and have a longer shelf life.

Organic cosmetics often are not all they claim to be. In some instances only one or two ingredients are natural products. These are then combined with synthetics—as in any standard cosmetic product.

One genuine difference between organic and nonorganic cosmetics is the greater danger of microbiological contamination in the organic products to which no preservatives have been added. For this reason, many such cosmetics are refrigerated.

LANOLIN IN COSMETICS

Many of today's cosmetics incorporate lanolin. What is lanolin, and does it provide any additional benefits? Is it safe?

Lanolin is the wool fat secreted from the sebaceous (oil) glands of sheep. It adheres to wool fibers and is extracted for commercial use by various means.

Lanolin has been used in ointments for many years because of its emulsifying and emollient properties; it makes ointments spread and adhere better when used in proper concentrations.

Some dermatologists consider lanolin a sensitizer, causing allergic skin reactions. Others believe that because lanolin sensitizes only a small percentage of users, its potential in this regard is not enough to cause concern. One must also recognize that the quality of lanolin available has been improved considerably over the years. Newer lanolin fractions and derivatives improve ointments and cosmetics even more than ordinary lanolin and are less likely to sensitize.

In addition to enhancing the emollient effect of creams and ointments, lanolin helps prevent excessive dryness of the skin and decreases the drying properties of detergent shampoos (but also reduces their cleansing power).

Lanolin will not prevent or cure wrinkles, stop hair loss or produce curly locks. It is a useful product, but not magic.

With decreasing world markets for wool, lanolin is becoming less available and synthetic substitutes are beginning to appear in the marketplace. It is still too early to pass judgment on these lanolin substitutes.

BREATH FRESHENERS

My teenaged daughter and her friends are using aerosol breath fresheners. Is there any danger?

These breath fresheners contain flavoring, artificial sweeteners, water, and alcohol. They are usually "metered," which means that only a small amount is expressed with each activation of the discharge button. The propellants themselves are similar to those used in all standard aerosol medications and food products. Regular and repeated use of this type of breath freshener poses no hazard. The amount of alcohol deposited on the tongue or membranes of the mouth is approximately one drop of an alcoholic beverage or mixed drink. Most conventional mouthwashes contain from 10 percent to 70 percent alcohol before dilution with water. Although misuse of some aerosol products to achieve drug-simulated effects has been reported, breath-freshener aerosol packages are too small to present such a hazard.

AUTOMATIC FACE CLEANSERS

Lately I've seen quite a few ads for automatic face cleansers. Some have attachments for massage and different brushes for gentle and deep cleansing. Are they safe?
Automatic face cleansers will not harm normal skin—but they won't cleanse it any better than a washcloth, soap, and water. Any device or abrasive skin preparation can only clean the surface of the skin, so be skeptical of claims for "superdeep-pore" cleansing.

If you have acne or excessively dry skin, automatic or manual complexion brushes can cause irritation, redness, and scaling. Even if you have normal skin, excessive or too vigorous use of these devices can lead to problems.

Brushes for "deep" cleansing are more likely to cause irritation than the softer ones for "gentle" cleansing. A facial massage temporarily increases blood flow to the skin, but produces no lasting effect.

ARTIFICIAL FINGERNAILS

Are any dangers associated with wearing false fingernails?
There are two types of artificial fingernails and either type can cause problems:

(1). Preformed artificial nails are made from synthetic materials of "secret" composition. They are attached to the natural nails with adhesive or simply pressed on, and then filed to shape. The adhesive used to attach the nails may cause an allergic reaction of the skin surrounding the nails. The artificial nails may also cause nail damage. If they are left on for more than a few days, the natural nails will soften and lift off because moisture accumulates under the impermeable plastics.

(2). Artificial nails that are formed on natural nails are made of plastic acrylic materials and have been associated with many reactions. These products consist of a liquid acrylic monomer (methyl methacrylate) and a powder polymer (polymethyl methacrylate) that are mixed together to form a polymerized, thick, viscous preparation that is brushed over a mold placed around the natural nail. The preparation may be used to form a complete artificial nail or a partial nail that covers the tip of the natural nail. The preparation hardens at room temperature within a few minutes to form an artificial nail that is firmly attached to the natural nail and "grows" with the natural nail, having a life that is claimed to be at least four weeks.

Acrylic nail preparations have produced many cases of allergic contact dermatitis of the skin. In addition, these artificial nails may cause painful inflammation and swelling of the soft tissue around the nail (a condition called paronychia) and separation of the natural nail from the nail bed (a condition called onychia). These conditions can be extremely painful and difficult to treat. Treatment of onychia is complicated by the fact that once the acrylic nail has hardened it is practically impossible to remove. The throbbing, swollen, painful nail is encased in a rigid plastic armor. Ice cold compresses may afford some relief, and strong sedation may have to be prescribed by a physician for several days. The nail may not return to its normal condition for several months.

ANTIPERSPIRANTS

> How do different kinds of antiperspirants compare in effectiveness? I am particularly interested in dry aerosol antiperspirants.

None of the presently available products will completely stop perspiration flow—nor is this desirable. The secretion of sweat is an essential function of the skin, important for temperature regulation and water metabolism of the body.

BRAND-NAME GUIDE TO DEODORANTS AND ANTIPERSPIRANTS

INGREDIENTS: BRANDS:*	Antiperspirants							Deodorants		
	Aluminum Chloride	Aluminum Chlorhydroxide	Zirconyl Hydroxychloride	Basic Aluminum Formate	Sodium Aluminum Lactate	Aluminum Sulfate	Methylbenzethonium Chloride	Triclosan	Zinc Phenolsulfonate	Cetyl Trimethyl Ammonium Bromide
CREAMS										
Arrid	•	•								
Avon										•
Fresh	•				•					
Mitchum	•	•								
Secret		•	•							
ROLL-ONS										
Arrid						•	•			
Avon		•								•
Ban		•								
Five-Day		•								
Mitchum	•	•						•		
Secret		•	•							
AEROSOLS										
Arrid Deodorant									•	
Arrid Extra Dry		•								
Light Powder and Extra Dry		•								
Dry Ban		•								
Ultra Ban	•	•								
Ultra Ban Powder Spray		•								
Calm II		•								
Dial Deodorant								•		
Dial Antiperspirant		•								
Fresh		•								
Manpower Deodorant									•	
Manpower Antiperspirant		•								
Mennen Deodorant									•	
Mennen Antiperspirant		•								
Mitchum Antiperspirant	•	•								
Right Guard Deodorant								•		
Right Guard Antiperspirant		•								
Secret Spray Deodorant									•	
Secret Spray Antiperspirant		•	•							
Soft Dri		•								
Stay Dri		•						•		

NOTE—The unscented forms of many of these products contain the same active ingredients.

*This list is representative of nationally available products. No attempt was made to list every brand.

The degree of perspiration control provided by different antiperspirant products may vary from 5 to 40 percent. Creams and roll-ons generally give greater protection than aerosol products. A product must reduce perspiration at least 20 to 25 percent to be considered a true antiperspirant. Products that do not control perspiration but do control body odor are termed deodorants.

According to one study, a leading roll-on antiperspirant reduced perspiration by 37 percent, a leading wet aerosol by only 5 percent, and a leading dry aerosol by about 27 percent. Most antiperspirant preparations have deodorant properties; this fact accounts for the public's acceptance of the less effective antiperspirants. The choice of one type over another is largely a matter of personal preference for ease of application, antiperspirant power, and odor control.

Industry surveys indicate that about 50 percent of consumers prefer roll-on and cream products because they give better antiperspirant and odor protection and do not burn or sting, even though they are somewhat less convenient to use. The other 50 percent prefer aerosols because they are quick and easy to use, are not messy, and the applicator does not come in contact with the skin. Many people do object to the sticky, wet, cold, burning, stinging and/or irritating feeling of wet aerosol products and do not find them effective or long-lasting in control of perspiration and body odor.

Dry aerosol antiperspirants, which several companies have introduced, are supposed to overcome these objections to wet aerosols. Manufacturers claim that dry aerosol products are effective for longer periods of time than wet aerosols, although not as long as roll-ons. (See Chapter 18, "Perspiration and Body Odor," for additional information on this subject.)

4

Reactions to Cosmetics

SENSITIVITY TO LIPSTICK

My lips always seem to be dry and cracked. I have been told that I may be allergic to lipstick. Are there any lipsticks that will not cause such a reaction?

First, it's important to find out whether you actually are allergic to lipstick. If your lips become inflamed and irritated, you may be sensitive (allergic) to one of the ingredients in your lipstick. Or you may be sensitive to some other substance; one girl's allergic reaction was provoked by her boy friend's mustache wax. Cheilitis (inflammation of the lips) may also be due to factors other than allergy; a physician can properly diagnose your condition.

Most lipsticks contain oil-wax mixtures, lanolin, a staining dye, perfume, and color pigments. Each of these substances except the pigments may cause an allergic reaction in some users. Should you be allergic to one of these substances, you may try specially formulated lipsticks from which one or more of these ingredients has been deleted. For instance, in addition to using special base ingredients and selected pigments, some manufacturers make "nonpermanent" lipsticks that do not contain the staining dye (a frequent offender). Other women may find that simply changing brands of ordinary lipstick will help them.

COSMETICS FOR SENSITIVE SKIN

I have a sensitive complexion that will not tolerate many cosmetics. Are any available that I can use safely?

Your dermatologist or allergist can best advise you about cosmetics that may solve your problem. Most manufacturers of cosmetics today have removed known irritating substances or, whenever possible, reduced their concentrations to a minimum; and most people can use these products safely.

Furthermore, some companies will supply your physician with the formulations of their products to aid in determining the cause of the reaction. Some companies also make available testing kits that can be used by your physician in determining whether you have a specific reaction to any one substance in the formula. If you are found to be sensitive to a particular substance, these firms will cooperate with you and your physician in providing formulations free of the offending components.

BROWN SPOTS FROM PERFUMES, AFTER-SHAVE LOTIONS

Recently when I returned from an afternoon at the beach, I noticed brown spots on my neck. My doctor told me they were caused by my perfume and would eventually disappear. Isn't there any treatment?

A number of perfumes contain ingredients called photosensitizers, which enhance the normal effect of ultraviolet light on the skin. Oil of bergamot, present in several perfumes, is considered such a photosensitizer. These ingredients may produce increased pigmentation (brown spots) where the perfume has been applied if the user is exposed to the sun shortly thereafter. Similar reactions to some after-shave lotions and men's colognes have been observed. This type of spotty pigmentation is known as "berlock dermatitis." While this reaction may be cosmetically disturbing, it is not serious.

There is no effective treatment, and the pigmentation generally persists for some time. It may be possible to camouflage the spots with masking cosmetics. Further use of the offending products on areas that may be exposed to sunlight and/or exposure of the pigmented area to sunlight should be avoided. These products may be used on covered areas, at night and during the winter (minimum sun) months.

SENSITIVITY TO PERFUME

Can you help me obtain ingredient information on a popular perfume to which I am allergic? When I wear this perfume or even come in contact with others who are wearing it, I have a severe allergic reaction. I wrote to the manufacturer, but all I learned was that the perfume does not contain any of the things to which I know I am allergic (as a result of tests I had as a child). My doctor has given me some medication to take in emergencies, but I would like to find out to which ingredients in the perfume I am allergic so that I can avoid these ingredients in the future.

Obtaining a list of ingredients for the perfume would probably be of little practical value to you. Perfumes are quite complex mixtures of essences and fixatives, a fact that makes allergy testing for these substances difficult. In addition, an allergic response can result from the combination of two or more ingredients, which tests with individual ingredients will not disclose. Since the number of potential ingredient combinations is so large, testing them is not practical.

A remote possibility is that the particular perfume (or ingredient in the perfume) is producing reactions in so many people that one of two things will happen: (1) the problem will be brought to the firm's attention by a large volume of complaint letters, or (2) consumers will no longer purchase the product, forcing the company to either reformulate or discontinue it.

You know you must avoid at least one specific perfume, but we are unable to advise you how to avoid the offending ingredient in other perfumes (this manufacturer's or someone else's). At present there is little demand to list all perfume ingredients on the perfume label. Some brands of cosmetics do come in essentially unscented forms, and this information is found on the label. So you yourself must determine—by trial and error—which perfumes and cosmetics you can use.

Since you have no control over the perfumes other people purchase or use, all you can do is what you are already doing— avoid contact with those wearing perfumes that provoke any allergic reaction in you. Seek out open, well-ventilated areas and avoid small, crowded, poorly ventilated places to reduce exposure to possible allergens. Your physician has already provided you with medication to use in emergency situations.

REACTIONS TO EYELINERS

Can eyeliner pencil be applied to the eyelid inside the lashes, or is this harmful?

The use of eyeliner pencil, mascara, and eye shadow to highlight the eyes is currently very popular. Some women apply eyeliner to the upper (and lower) borders of the eyelids inside the lashes, rather than to the surface of the eyelid behind the lashes.

According to a report by an eye specialist, this may lead to various problems, including permanent pigmentation of the conjunctiva (the membrane lining the lids and covering the eyes), moderate redness, itching, tearing and blurring of vision. The physician examined fourteen women aged fifteen to forty who used eyeliner pencil: many of them had all or several of the complaints mentioned above.

In a report the doctor urged: "When they must use a cosmetic around their eyes, women should be urged to confine it to the lashes and to the skin external to them. . . . I have not seen a patient who used cosmetics inside the lashes who had completely normal conjunctivas."

EYE INFECTIONS FROM MASCARA

Is it true that you can get an eye infection from using borrowed mascara?

Borrowing and lending mascara, eyeliner, and other eye makeup has led to at least one epidemic of the severe eye infection trachoma, according to a report by a California physician. The outbreak of trachoma resulted from schoolgirls borrowing eyeliner pencils; the practice of borrowing and lending mascara and other cosmetics should be discouraged.

BACTERIAL CONTAMINATION OF EYE MAKEUP

I have read that eye cosmetics are contaminated with bacteria. Is there any risk in the use of such products?

Most eye cosmetics, like other cosmetic products, are manufactured in clean, modern facilities. "Good Manufacturing Practices," a set of production procedures developed by industry and government, prevail in essentially all cosmetics manufacturing plants. While greater care is taken in the manufacture of cosmetics for the eye area, there is no attempt (and no need) to sterilize these products. Few, if any, reach the consumer in a state that poses the risk of infection.

Major contamination occurs during application of the product by the user. Microorganisms picked up from the user's skin by the brush, applicator, or finger are transferred to the product. Since most contaminating organisms are those from the user's own skin, it is unlikely that they represent a serious health hazard. However, to prevent their growth to numbers that would pose a threat to health, manufacturers incorporate preservative agents in their products. These preservatives, given a few hours in which to exert their influence (i.e., between consecutive uses of the eye cosmetic), are able to reduce the number of microorganisms.

Selection of the preservative agent is made on the basis of its safety in uses around the eye as well as on its antimicrobial (germ-fighting) activity. The concentration of the preservative used is selected to assure chemical safety as well as microbiological safety, and is related to normal use patterns for such products. Only a very strong preservative in high concentrations could maintain a cosmetic product at near sterile levels, especially shortly after use. Since such strong preservatives in the necessary concentrations pose safety problems of a different type, their use in eye cosmetics is not desirable.

To avoid infections, don't borrow or lend eye cosmetics, since by doing so you defeat the built-in safeguards. When purchasing eye makeup, select packaging that will help minimize contamination. For example, buy tubes and self-applicators instead of open containers or those that must be moistened before application. Immediately stop using any product that causes irritation, and visit a physician if irritation persists. Wash your hands before using eye cosmetics and avoid use of saliva to moisten cosmetics.

Finally, remember that special care must be taken in the application of eye makeup. Apply the makeup at home, not in an automobile or any other moving vehicle. A number of serious eye infections have been reported in which the initiating event appears to have been a scratch on the cornea caused by the applicator brush.

EYE DAMAGE FROM SPRAYS

Is it harmful for hair spray to come in contact with the eyes?

Yes. All aerosol preparations—including hair sprays, deodorants, and less frequently used preparations such as nasal sprays and insecticides—should be kept away from the eyes.

As the use of aerosol preparations increases, so does the number of eye injuries that physicians observe among users.

The injuries are caused by tiny chemical particles that leave the nozzle of the spray can at high speed. The particles, which are smaller than dust specks, fan out and strike a large area. They may become imbedded in the cornea of the eye, causing redness and irritation. Most injuries are minor and may clear up in a week or more. However, some particles that are deeply imbedded may cause permanent discoloration.

There is some danger that freezing resulting from rapid evaporation of the aerosol propellants will damage sensitive eye tissues. Sprays also may interfere with the wearing of contact lenses. One physician reported that a number of patients who were unable to wear contact lenses because of the pain they caused were able to do so comfortably after they stopped using sprays and the injuries healed—injuries of which the patients had not been aware.

When using any spray preparation, be careful to protect your eyes. Also be careful not to accidentally spray anyone who might be standing nearby.

FINGERNAIL-HARDENING PREPARATIONS

Can formaldehyde cause skin reactions when used as a nail hardener?

Skin reactions to formaldehyde exposure are well known; this chemical is both an irritant and a sensitizer. Reactions may be increasing in frequency as a result of greater public contact with formaldehyde in various forms. For instance, fabrics are sometimes treated with formaldehyde resins to provide a permanent press finish, and clothing made from these fabrics occasionally causes skin reactions.

In recent years, products to prevent the nails from chipping, fragmenting, and peeling have become popular. Some of these products contain formaldehyde or ingredients that gradually release formaldehyde. Reactions to such preparations have included discoloration, bleeding under the nails, pain, dryness, and loosening or even loss of the nails. The cuticle and surrounding skin have also been affected. Reactions may persist for several weeks or months.

While formaldehyde nail hardeners may be helpful for nail hardening, the potential user should realize that a risk is involved. If a reaction occurs, a physician should be consulted for treatment. Brittle nails are discussed in more detail in Chapter 17, "Hand, Nail, and Foot Problems."

BLOTCHY SKIN

I have been using a "skin-tone cream" containing hydroquinone that is advertised to lighten, brighten, and soften the skin of dark-skinned people. Now my skin is all blotchy. What can I do to make my skin look normal again? Is there any other product that will safely lighten and brighten my skin?

Hydroquinone is a moderately effective drug when used to treat excess pigmentation caused by disease of or injury to the skin. It is considerably less effective as a depigmenting agent on normal skin.

The response of normal black skin to hydroquinone treatment for depigmentation depends on the amount of pigment present. Lighter black skin is partly depigmented, while no depigmentation of darker black skin is observed. After treatment is stopped, repigmentation almost always occurs. Some hydroquinone drugs are powerful depigmenting agents and can produce blotchiness and other undesirable effects when not properly used; these products have limited medical usefulness and should be used only under close medical supervision.

It is difficult to make an accurate prediction concerning the uneven pigmentation you mention. So much depends on its cause. While an uneven pigmentation may be due to the use of hydroquinone cream, a number of diseases can produce uneven pigmentation. Blotchy skin color may also be inherited. To make your skin look normal again, the best advice would be to leave it alone completely, using only ordinary soap-and-water washing and, if your skin is very dry, a simple cold cream.

Many people who use "skin-tone creams" are really employing them for their emollient or skin-softening effects. Such effects can easily be obtained with simple, inexpensive cold creams and lubricating creams.

At present there is no readily available, safe, simple, effective way to significantly lighten normal skin coloration.

DISCOLORATION FROM SKIN BLEACHES

I have been using a bleaching cream advertised to remove age spots from the hands. Now I have developed a bluish-black discoloration on my hands that looks worse than the age spots. Is there any way to get rid of the discoloration?

Continuous, long-term use of bleaching preparations that contain ammoniated mercury as the active ingredient (for more than a few months at a time) may cause a skin discoloration such as you describe. Mercury from the cream is deposited in the skin, and the discoloration is permanent. Mercury compounds can also produce internal adverse effects.

For these and other reasons, in 1974 the Federal Food and Drug Administration banned the use of mercury compounds in nonprescription products except eye cosmetics, where they can be used in small concentrations as a preservative. Thus, you should no longer be able to purchase bleaching creams containing ammoniated mercury. It would be a good idea to dispose of any you may have on hand.

LOSS OF EYELASHES

I wear mascara on my eyelashes every day. When I wash it off, I lose two or three eyelashes from each eye. Is the mascara causing these eyelashes to fall out? Will they grow back?

Mascara does not cause eyelashes to fall out, although loose ones may come out during the application or removal of mascara. You cannot prevent loose eyelashes from falling out, but it is reassuring to know that normally they will grow back.

It is natural for a few eyelash hairs to fall out daily. This occurs because human hair—eyelashes, eyebrows, body hair, and scalp hair—grows in cycles. After an eyelash hair grows for about six months, it begins a resting period in which the hair stops growing and separates from the root. The hair then moves slowly upward and is easily dislodged by washing, rubbing the eyes, or applying or removing mascara. After the resting phase a new hair forms in the follicle, initiating a new growth cycle. If the old hair is still in place, the new hair will push it out. Each hair has its own growth cycle. Generally, only a small percentage of hairs are in the resting phase and being shed at any one time, so the loss usually is not obvious.

5

Cosmetics — Miscellaneous

WHICH BRAND IS BEST?

In purchasing a cosmetic product, which brand should I select? With so many different products available, it is difficult to know which is best.

Since we have no program for evaluating various products, we are not in a position to recommend specific brands of cosmetics.

However, you may be interested to know that measuring the differences among brands of many cosmetic products, such as cold cream or face powder, is often difficult because they are basically so much alike. Selection of one brand over another usually depends solely on personal preference for such qualities as shade, scent, texture, or even package design.

When a company markets a product on a national basis with anticipation of large consumer acceptance, the product is made as trouble-free as possible to help it gain wide acceptance. However, a locally sold product may be just as "safe."

Price is not always the best guide to quality in cosmetics. Several low-priced products have proven, through years of satisfactory use, to compare favorably with similar but more expensive items.

Each cosmetic product should be evaluated on an individual basis. Many women are willing to try a new product of a familiar brand line, on the assumption that responsible manufacturers are interested in preserving the quality of that line. Such an assumption is no substitute for personal experimentation with individual products.

COSMETICS AND THE LAW

Do the provisions of the Food, Drug, and Cosmetic Act protect the consumer's health adequately as far as cosmetic products are concerned?

The principal difficulty in answering this question is that the word "cosmetic" means different things to the consumer and to the government. Both the cosmetics industry and the government share some responsibility for this.

A simplified legal definition is that a product is a cosmetic when its sole purpose is adornment; it is a drug if it has any effect on the structure or function of the skin or any other organ.

Today there is a trend toward "medicated cosmetics," products to which some medically active ingredients have been added. Legally, most "medicated cosmetics" are drugs.

The manufacturer of a cosmetic product has only two legal obligations: (1) to carry out enough tests to assure that the product appears safe, and (2) to label it properly. The requirements for drugs are considerably more restrictive. Since medicated cosmetics are packaged as cosmetics and are marketed in the cosmetics sections of drug and department stores, the consumer is under the impression that such products are "true" cosmetics and may not pay adequate attention to the labels and instructions for use.

Many products have the approval of the Federal Food and Drug Administration for use as directed on the label. Most consumers don't realize that in a number of cases these directions refer to maximum safe usage; there is little to alert the consumer to possible hazards of unrestricted use. Among consumer products, legal requirements for labeling of all cosmetics are relatively lax and do little to insure the public health and interest. New federal regulations will effect needed improvements in this area.

Since legal distinctions between cosmetics and medicated cosmetics are sometimes finely drawn, the best advice for consumers is that they read all informational material supplied with these products. This includes statements made on the container itself, on the carton in which it is packaged and in any accompanying printed material. In the eyes of the law, all of this constitutes labeling.

COSMETIC INGREDIENT LABELING

Is it true that ingredients in cosmetics must be listed on the label? I recently bought some cosmetics and this information was not listed.

The government issued a regulation on March 3, 1975, that requires cosmetics manufacturers to list ingredients on the labels. However, you should not expect to see all cosmetics labeled in this way for a while.

In a mass-production industry such as the cosmetics industry, changes affecting all products produced by every firm are difficult to bring about quickly and economically. Large stocks of labels must be available to meet production requirements, and orders for such labels are placed well in advance of need. Thus in its present form the regulation requires only that all new labels ordered after March 3, 1976, contain appropriate ingredient information. The regulation further requires that only labels with appropriate ingredient information will be used in the identification of all products manufactured after September 3, 1976.

Some companies have begun to label their products with ingredient information. Most have waited for more clarification to be certain of the requirements before ordering new labeling. Delays experienced in bringing these labeling regulations to the present stage indicate the complexity of some of the problems related to shortages of product ingredients, as well as problems of labeling small packages such as lipsticks and eye products. With time, all cosmetic products will be appropriately labeled with ingredient information.

USEFULNESS OF COSMETIC-INGREDIENT LABEL-ING

Will cosmetic-ingredient labeling be useful to the average consumer?

Cosmetic-ingredient labeling will provide the consumer with some information, although fragrance and flavors will not be identified.

The names of many individual cosmetic ingredients will appear strange—and may indeed be meaningless without the assistance of a cosmetic-ingredient dictionary.

It is expected that in the future more and more consumers who experience reactions to cosmetic products will be able, through appropriate medical evaluation, to determine which ingredient in a particular cosmetic was responsible for the reaction. By reading cosmetic labels before purchasing, the consumer will be able to avoid further exposure to this ingredient.

Ingredient listing will indicate only relative concentrations of ingredients, will usually not indicate ingredient quality, and will not indicate the care that has been utilized in formulating, manufacturing, or testing the product. Ingredient listing as required in the present regulation will therefore be of little value in comparison shopping.

DOOR-TO-DOOR COSMETICS

A saleswoman called at my home to sell me a line of cosmetics unknown to me. She said these products are not available in stores. Would such cosmetics be safe to use? Why aren't they available in stores?

All cosmetics sold in interstate commerce, through retail outlets or door-to-door, must comply with the same federal standards. These standards help to assure the consumer that the products are safe.

Several lines of cosmetics are sold door-to-door instead of through retail outlets. Some "direct-selling" firms have been in business for many years and have established a reputation for quality products. In fact, the country's largest cosmetics firm uses this sales approach.

Of course, when purchasing any cosmetic you should use common sense in evaluating claims made by the salesperson and in the advertising materials. Exaggerated claims of superiority should be viewed with healthy skepticism. For instance, the addition of "extra" or "exotic" ingredients (such as turtle oil, strawberry extract or mysterious chemicals) rarely serves any purposes beneficial to the consumer.

AIRBORNE COSMETICS

I've never heard of anyone hesitating to take aerosol cosmetics aboard a plane, but now have been told that it's illegal. Is this true?

Until a couple of years ago it was true—at least theoretically. According to Federal Aviation Administration regulations, passengers had to wrap and label as "dangerous" any aerosol product (hair spray, shaving cream, etc.) or flammable liquid (perfume, medicine containing alcohol, etc.) carried on board.

Most travelers, however, were probably unaware of the ruling, and simply tossed their toiletry and medical items into a carry-on bag without a second thought. Now the FAA says it's all right, as long as certain weight limitations are met. Aerosol containers may be of any size, but all other items must weigh less than 16 ounces, and the total, including that in carry-on luggage and checked baggage, must not exceed 75 ounces.

HYPOALLERGENIC COSMETICS

What is the present status of hypoallergenic cosmetics?
It became evident about thirty-five years ago that cosmetic products were producing allergic reactions in some users. A few manufacturers therefore began to produce cosmetic lines from which known sensitizing agents were omitted. These manufacturers published the formulations of their products and provided physicians who requested them with supplies of individual ingredients for sensitization tests as well as with specially formulated products.

The term "hypoallergenic" was coined to differentiate these cosmetics from others available at the time. This term, it was hoped, would indicate that products so labeled were less likely to produce allergic reactions in consumers. Since in those days a large number of reactions were correctly or incorrectly associated with perfume ingredients, most hypoallergenic cosmetics became available in unscented as well as scented formulations. There have been few changes in the policies of the manufacturers of these specially formulated cosmetics since that time.

A significant change has occurred, however, in the formulations used by manufacturers of major brands of cosmetic products. These manufacturers and their suppliers of raw materials came to realize that it was in their best interest to eliminate ingredients likely to cause a significant number of allergic reactions among consumers.

Thus, at present we find little distinction among established cosmetic products concerning their sensitization potential. Reactions to cosmetic products are relatively rare, occur with so-called hypoallergenic cosmetics as well as with those not so labeled, and involve individual idiosyncrasies to specific ingredients. If a patient who experiences an adverse reaction to a particular cosmetic product switches from her normal brand to a hypoallergenic brand, her problem might be solved.

However, the same result will probably be obtained if she switches to another standard brand of cosmetic products.

In other words, it may be said that: (1) ingredients most likely to cause sensitization have been eliminated from most cosmetic products, and (2) allergic reactions may occur when so-called hypoallergenic cosmetics are used, since there is no method known by which a nonallergenic cosmetic can be produced.

A small difference between the original hypoallergenic cosmetic brands and other products is that many manufacturers of hypoallergenic cosmetics usually are a bit quicker to make available to physicians information and services concerning their products. These services make it possible for a physician to identify more rapidly the allergen involved in any given case and to adopt an appropriately modified formulation.

REFRIGERATING COSMETICS

Is it true that cosmetic creams and lotions should be kept refrigerated to avoid spoiling?

Refrigeration is not necessary for the majority of commercially available cosmetics. These products contain preservatives that inhibit the growth of microorganisms that get into them during normal use. A properly preserved cosmetic cream or lotion is to some degree self-sterilizing and quite safe to use for a reasonably long time.

The only cosmetic creams and lotions that require refrigeration are those that do not contain preservatives—homemade cosmetics or those made from organic ingredients only (fruits, vegetables, various plants, or dairy products).

COSMETIC POISONING

I understand that cosmetic products account for some poisonings. Would warning labels help prevent these poisonings?

Yes, warning labels probably would be helpful. According to statistics from the Poison Control Program of the Canadian Food and Drug Directorate, 5 percent of all poisonings in 1969 involved cosmetic products. Of these, 90 percent were "accidents" with children aged four and younger.

In 90 percent of the followed up poisonings of preschool children, one or both parents were caring for the child at the time of the accident.

In 69 percent of all poisoning cases (where this information was available), the product was in its original container at the time of ingestion, and in 26 percent the original container carried a warning label.

Warning labels won't do the children any good, but they might motivate parents to make a deliberate effort to keep these products inaccessible to youngsters. The labels could also carry first-aid instructions, telling parents and other adults what to do if the product is swallowed.

COSMETIC SAFETY INFORMATION

Is it possible to obtain information concerning the relative safety of various cosmetic products?
This information is not readily available. Many cosmetic firms conduct premarketing evaluations when a new product is introduced. The marketing firms can use this information to improve cosmetic formulas when the need arises. Unfortunately, however, safety information derived from the tests and evaluations is usually available only to the sponsoring firms.

Many reactions to cosmetic products are mild irritations, and most consumers simply switch products until they find one suitable for themselves. More serious reactions require medical attention, but the physician and patient are usually more interested in improving the patient's condition than in reporting the adverse reaction.

If all cosmetic reactions were reported to the manufacturer, the Food and Drug Administration, or the American Medical Association, both consumer and industry would benefit. To date, established statistics concerning cosmetic reactions are not available, although attempts to obtain better statistics are under way. It is difficult to ascribe a reaction to a cosmetic (or a drug) unless the problem has been properly evaluated by a knowledgeable physician. Also, reactions due to inappropriate use of products (swallowing by children) or injuries resulting from accidents with containers should be distinguished from reactions that result from normal use of products.

Part II
HAIR

6

Hair Dyes and Bleaches

TYPES OF HAIR-COLORING PREPARATIONS

What are the different types of hair-coloring preparations?
The major types of hair-coloring products are (1) permanent oxidation dyes and toners, (2) semipermanent dyes, (3) temporary colors (acid rinses), (4) metallic dyes, (5) vegetable dyes, and (6) bleaches. A discussion of each type of preparation follows.

PERMANENT OXIDATION DYES

What are oxidation dyes? How effective are they?
Almost all professional hair coloring is done with dyes known as permanent, developed, or oxidation dyes. These are also the most popular hair colors for home use, because they are the only hair-coloring products that not only color hair quickly but produce all varieties of natural hair shades that are lasting and pleasing. All oxidation dyes require that the hair dye be mixed with an equal volume of developer (20-volume peroxide) immediately before using, because the principal ingredients are dye intermediates that form dyes only when mixed with a developer. Because this chemical reaction (oxidation) must take place within the hair to produce desired results, the dye and developer must be mixed just before use.

Professional products may be applied with a brush, swab, or applicator using the technique known as "parting and sectioning." Most products for home use, and some professional products, are applied as "shampoo-in" hair colors.

Because the new color is formed inside the hair, these dyes produce a fairly permanent effect. This is both a strength and a weakness. The user doesn't have to worry about the color washing out, but if she is not satisfied with the effect, the color is difficult to remove.

Oxidation dyes will lighten the hair, but, unless the hair is prebleached, the degree of lightening usually is limited to no more than two or three shades. Most brands include in the package directions a clear, concise explanation of what can be expected. The directions will indicate that if your hair is color X it can go no lighter than color Y.

The package directions will also say that a color test should be performed on a lock of hair. This test will indicate just what color to expect from your hair in its present condition. It is important to carry out this test, since unexpected color reactions may result when hair is damaged or has been dyed previously with a metallic dye.

The accumulated experience with oxidation dyes is so great that the results are more predictable than with newer dyes. Such reliability may be a real asset to the user. The safety aspects of these products are discussed later in this chapter.

INTERVAL BETWEEN DYEINGS

How frequently can hair be dyed?
An interval of three to four weeks is necessary between dyeings. More frequent applications may result in overfragility and loss of normal texture.

Temporary acid color rinses or color sticks can be used to touch up untinted roots that begin to show. These preparations are water-soluble and are easily removed by regular shampooing.

Don't try to change your hair color too frequently or too radically—for example, from dark brown to blond or red. You may get green hair instead, or your damaged, more fragile hair may break off close to the scalp. One of the large cosmetic firms indicates that the greatest number of complaints are received from people who have tried at home to change the color of their hair drastically and/or too frequently. Drastic color changes require professional techniques—and even then damage to the hair cannot always be prevented.

SEMIPERMANENT DYES

What are semipermanent hair-coloring preparations? How long will the color last?

Semipermanent dyes are organic dyes that do not require an oxidizing agent (developer) to color hair. Thus they do not require mixing prior to use. These products are called semipermanent because they produce substantial color changes lasting through several shampoos. According to brand, they may be applied as shampoos or as rinses following shampooing.

Semipermanent dyes can produce an immediate or gradual color change, depending on the method of application. If the dye is left on the hair for a long time (20 to 30 minutes or the full time indicated in the package directions), full-color effects are immediate. If the dye is left on for a short time (5 to 10 minutes), only a small color effect is produced; but repeated applications at weekly intervals will deepen the color to that achieved in the longer, single application. Because color change is not so noticeable, the gradual method may be preferred by those who have gray hair and/or are self-conscious about dyeing their hair. Semipermanent dyes used in this manner should not be confused with metallic dyes, which also produce a gradual color change. (Metallic dyes are discussed later in this chapter.)

The disadvantage of semipermanent hair colors is that as yet they do not reproduce the dark brown and black natural shades that can be obtained from oxidation dyes. They perform well in light shades; will brighten "mousy" hair, and will color partially gray hair.

AEROSOL HAIR DYES

Recently I have seen advertisements for an aerosol hair dye. How does this dye differ from other hair dyes?
Aerosol foam hair dyes either are permanent oxidation or semipermanent dyes, and produce the same color effects on the hair as their nonaerosol counterparts. Aerosol foam dyes of the semipermanent type differ from similar nonaerosol dyes only in the form of packaging and the method of application; the dye is packaged in an aerosol container from which it is sprayed directly onto the hair as a foam. Aerosol foam dyes of the permanent oxidation type differ from nonaerosol dyes not only in packaging and application, but also in method of mixing before use. The rest of this answer is devoted to these permanent dyes.

All oxidation dyes require that the hair dye be mixed with an equal volume of developer (20-volume hydrogen peroxide) immediately before using. This is necessary because the principal ingredients form dyes only when mixed with a developer, and the chemical reaction (called oxidation) must take place within the hair to produce the desired results.

In nonaerosol oxidation dyes, the hair dye and developer are packaged in two separate containers, and the contents must be mixed by the user. In permanent aerosol hair dyes, the hair dye and developer are packaged in separate compartments inside the aerosol can and are mixed automatically as the product is dispensed.

Aerosol hair dye was made possible by development of an aerosol can with two separate compartments (a plastic container within the metal container) and a valve construction and dispensing mechanism that automatically mixes measured amounts of the contents of each container as the product is dispensed.

In addition to their convenience, aerosol hair dyes may be more economical. All of the dye and developer of permanent nonaerosol hair dyes is mixed together before using, and any unused dye must be discarded. Since aerosol preparations are mixed as they are dispensed, any of the product remaining in the aerosol container can be retained for later use.

On the other hand, aerosol hair dyes will not color hair correctly if dye and developer are not mixed in proper proportions as they are dispensed. Improper mixture can occur if the valve dispenser malfunctions, or if the ratio of the two ingredients changes as the aerosol container empties.

SAFETY ASPECTS OF OXIDATION AND SEMIPERMANENT DYES

Are any hazards associated with using oxidation or semipermanent hair-coloring preparations?

Oxidation dyes are more sensitizing than most other hair colorings, although today the incidence of sensitization compared to the number of applications is very low. "Sensitizing" means developing an allergy. If the dye is applied to a sensitized person, a skin irritation (dermatitis) develops. This can be mild or severe, local or general, depending on how intense the sensitization is and how much skin contact occurs with the dye. The usual case of hair dye dermatitis results in considerable swelling around the eyes; redness and crusting of the skin of the face, ears, and neck; and itching and discomfort.

The long-range effects of semipermanent dyes are not known, since these products are relatively new; however, they appear to be quite safe. The incidence of allergic reactions is very low, but the products are considered sensitizers.

Federal legislation requires that all oxidation and semipermanent dyes carry a warning on the label that a patch test must be performed before each application of the dye. Instructions for performing this test are included in each package.

The warning statement will read: "Caution—this product contains ingredients that may cause skin irritation in certain individuals, and a preliminary test according to accompanying directions should first be made. This product may not be used for dyeing eyelashes or eyebrows; to do so may cause blindness." This statement and the package directions should be read and followed carefully every time one of these products is used. Sensitivity may not develop until after a product has been used many times. People cannot be desensitized to these dyes, and repeated applications may increase the degree of sensitivity. Thus, a person who has become allergic to one of these dyes should never use the dye again, as it may result in a violent contact dermatitis. If a sensitized person has any questions, a dermatologist or an allergist should be consulted.

The person who has developed a sensitivity to an oxidation or semipermanent dye may be able to use metallic dye safely, although the cosmetic results will be less satisfactory.

PATCH TESTING PROCEDURE

How is the hair dye patch test carried out? How significant are the results?

The patch test involves application of a small amount of dye, mixed as for actual use, either to the skin behind the ear or on the inside of the arm at the elbow. This test area should remain uncovered and untouched by eyeglasses, combs, or other objects for 24 to 48 hours. If redness, burning, itching, blisters, or eruptions appear at this site during that time, the reaction is positive and under no circumstances should the dye be used.

No reaction simply indicates that the person is not sensitive to that dye at that particular time and under those conditions. It cannot be predicted which persons will become sensitive at a later date, especially if the brand or color of the dye is changed. Furthermore, manufacturers sometimes change the ingredients in a preparation.

The user also changes and may become allergic to the (unchanged) dye at any time. (This is similar to the case of a person who contracts hay fever at age thirty, even though he or she has lived in the same area and been exposed to ragweed all his or her life.) Scalp irritation due to disease, physical trauma, or chemical injury from hair and scalp products may predispose one to an allergy to dyes. This unrelated scalp irritation also may be misinterpreted as an allergy to the dye. Thus, it is necessary to perform the skin test before each application of the dye to be certain that no allergenic sensitivity has developed.

WHEN TO PATCH TEST

I have my hair dyed regularly, but find it inconvenient to visit the beauty shop the day before to have a patch test that will determine whether I have become sensitive (allergic) to the hair dye. Can I have the patch test performed the week before, when I visit the beauty shop for a shampoo and set?

Yes. Even though a patch test is not always convenient, one must be performed before each and every application of hair dye. If you can't go in for a patch test a day or two beforehand, have it done the previous week.

The purpose of a patch test is to determine whether a person has been sensitized by the last application of hair dye. After the patch test is applied, 24 to 48 hours is required for the subject to react to the test material. Actually, a patch test performed a week before the hair dye application may be preferable because it allows adequate time (48 hours is better than 24) for the reaction to develop. If the area to which the patch test has been applied becomes red and itches, the patch test is positive and the client is now allergic to the hair dye. If the area remains unchanged, the patch test is negative and the client is not reactive to the hair dye at that particular time.

HAIR DYES FOR HOME USE WITHOUT PATCH TESTING

Is there a hair dye that I can use safely at home that does not require patch testing?

Yes, metallic salt and vegetable dyes and most temporary rinses can be used at home quite safely and do not require patch testing. However, they will produce a limited range of colors, none of which too closely resembles the natural color of hair.

METALLIC SALT DYES

What are the pros and cons of using metallic salt dyes?

Metallic salt dyes usually contain a lead compound. The salts undergo a chemical change to deposit a colored film along the hair shaft without penetration.

These preparations have several disadvantages from a cosmetic point of view. Since the coloring substance is deposited on the outside of the hair like a plating, the natural luster is obscured. Several applications of the metallic salt dye may be required to produce an appreciable change in hair coloring. Thus they are sometimes referred to as progressive dyes. Years ago, enterprising manufacturers exploited this deficiency by calling these products "hair-color restorers" to imply that color gradually would return to gray hair. This term finally was banned.

Another disadvantage is the limited number of available shades. (There is no shade selection.) These dyes tend to produce dark and intense colors rather than muted lighter shades, which are more becoming. In addition, metallic salt dyes may interfere with permanent waving.

On the other hand, these dyes are very easy to use at home. Self-conscious people, particularly men, use them in the hope that their associates will not realize they are dyeing their hair, since the color change is very gradual and is more likely to pass without notice.

Finally, these dyes are probably safer than any of the other types. Strong evidence indicates that metallic salts are not absorbed through intact skin; however, care should be exercised to prevent their contact with mucous membranes or skin lesions and to avoid accidental ingestion. There is little if any evidence that persons become allergically sensitized to metallic dyes as they do to organic dyes, although most metallic dyes carry a warning statement "for external use only" or "contains ingredients that may cause skin irritation."

Although the use of metallic salt dyes is limited today, several brands are available. (See the brand-name guide at end of chapter.)

VEGETABLE DYES

What are vegetables dyes? How do they compare with other hair dyes?

Vegetable dyes have probably been in use longer than any other hair dyes. Thousands of years of use have established their safety as well as their cosmetic limitations. Vegetable hair dyes once used but rarely, if ever, seen today include indigo, camomile, logwood, and walnut hull extract. All required lengthy application and produced only a limited number of hair shades that were seldom pleasing or uniform.

The only vegetable dye still employed to any extent is henna. Henna consists of the ground-up, dried leaves and stems of a shrub found in North Africa and the Near East. This powder is made into a paste with hot water and applied directly to the hair. Only a reddish color is produced, the intensity varying with the length of application. The chief virtue of henna is its safety; it has no apparent toxic qualities and almost never sensitizes.

DYE REMOVAL

I have been dyeing my hair, but no longer wish to continue. How can I remove the dye so that it won't be noticeable when my hair starts to grow?

Once hair has been colored with a permanent dye, there is no satisfactory method for removing the dye. New, undyed hair must be allowed to grow out.

Preparations known as color removers or "strippers" are available for removing some dyes from hair, but they should be applied only by a professional beautician. Bleach preparations that contain so-called "boosters" can also be used by beauticians to remove or considerably lighten permanent dyes. Bleaches are potentially less damaging than color removers, but damage may result from either method, especially if the hair is already damaged by overbleaching, overdyeing, or overprocessing from permanents.

DYEING GRAY HAIR

I have to dye my hair every two weeks to cover the gray. Is it safe to dye hair this often?

Assuming the dye is a permanent oxidation type, it should be used no more often than once every three weeks. More frequent use may damage hair or produce undesirable shades of color, unless great care is taken to dye only new growth. This may be a difficult task for the home user.

If the dye color is a very dark brown or black shade, a new growth of gray hair will be more noticeable than with a "softer" or lighter shade. Temporary rinses, shampoos, or color sticks help conceal new growth of gray hair between dyeings, and can be used safely as frequently as needed.

Of course, if your hair is now totally gray, you may want

to let the gray hair grow in. Then, if necessary, use one of the temporary or semipermanent colors that give highlights to gray hair or conceal yellow tones. Several brands are marketed specifically for this purpose. Most people consider well-groomed gray hair attractive.

TEMPORARY COLORS

What kind of coloring preparation can I use to tone down my gray hair? I don't wish to use a permanent dye.
You would probably find one of the temporary acid rinses satisfactory. These colors primarily add highlights, tone down gray or yellow hair, brighten faded hair and blend streaked hair. They cannot produce drastic changes in hair color. The rinses also contain mild organic acids that enable them to remove dulling soap film from hair in the same manner as vinegar or lemon rinses, and the color is easily removed by shampooing.

Color rinses are available in either dry or liquid form. The dyes used are for the most part acid dyes certified by the federal government for use in foods, drugs or cosmetics. Hair coloring preparations that contain synthetic organic dyes other than certified colors will carry a caution statement on the label like those required by law for oxidation and semipermanent dyes.

Liquid rinses are usually aqueous acid solutions of dyes, using harmless organic acids. The popular dry preparations consist of a crystalline organic acid in which the crystals are coated with dyes. In use, a small amount of the concentrate is dissolved in warm water and poured through the hair. When used in high concentrations the effect is not natural.

High-intensity temporary colors are also available in which the color can be removed by one shampoo. With these it is possible to impart deeper colors that will not rub off. Most products of this type are applied to the hair full strength and allowed to remain for 5 to 30 minutes for full color effect.

High-intensity temporary colors can produce varied hair color effects that can be changed at will. These rinses usually contain noncertified colors and will always carry a cautionary statement on the label.

HOW TO DISTINGUISH AMONG TYPES OF HAIR DYE

How can the consumer distinguish among various types of hair coloring preparations?

The consumer should be able to distinguish among various types of hair coloring preparations by carefully checking the labeling on the package.

The packaging of permanent oxidation dyes includes a cautionary statement, directions for patch testing, and an indication that the product provides permanent color. The dye and the developer are in separate containers that must be mixed prior to use, unless the product is an aerosol foam.

While semipermanent preparations also carry a cautionary statement and include directions for patch testing, the product does not require mixing prior to use, and there is an indication on the package that the results will last only for a few shampoos (generally four or five).

The packaging of temporary preparations always indicates that the color is temporary and can be removed by shampooing.

Metallic salt dyes are easy to distinguish from other types of dyes because they are the only dyes that offer no shade selection. Also, the directions will indicate that color develops progressively with each application. Henna, the only vegetable dye used to any extent, is usually listed as an ingredient on the package; thus, it is easily distinguished from metallic dyes.

As a further aid, a brand-name guide to nationally advertised hair coloring preparations is provided at the end of this chapter.

HAIR DYES FOR MEN

Hair dyes for men are being promoted as something new and different. Are any hazards associated with their use?
For many years, most hair dyes promoted for men were metallic salt dyes. In recent years, however, permanent oxidation dyes and semipermanent dyes identical to those marketed for women, but with more masculine brand names, have become available. See previous answers in this chapter for a discussion of the effects of these types of hair dyes.

NO INTERNAL REACTIONS TO HAIR DYES

Is it true that hair dyes can affect the mind or cause other serious internal problems?
Hair dyes, when used according to directions, are considered safe products. Certain types of hair dyes, such as permanent oxidation dyes and semipermanent dyes, may cause allergic skin reactions in some persons; however, no hair dye is known to cause serious internal reactions.

EYELASH DYES

My eyelashes are very light colored. Is there a dye that I can safely apply to make them more noticeable?
The only way to color eyelashes is with mascara. No other type of preparation should be used on eyelashes because of potential danger to the eye. Severe eye injury and even blindness may result from dyeing of eyelashes or eyebrows. If you want to further accentuate your eyelashes, wear false eyelashes.

PREBLEACHING AND TONERS

I want to change the color of my hair from brown to silvery blond. My hairdresser said this would require prebleaching and use of a toner. Please explain this technique.

If you desire to lighten your hair by more than two or three shades, prebleaching is required. In prebleaching, ammoniacal hydrogen peroxide mixed with a hair lightener is applied to the hair to bleach out much or all of the color. Prebleaching also increases the hair fibers' porosity so that the hair will absorb the toner that is ordinarily applied after bleaching. Toners are specially formulated oxidation or semipermanent dyes in pale blond shades that give a small amount of color to bleached hair. (See the exchange on toners later in this chapter.)

Because bleaching increases porosity and brittleness of the hair fibers, it can be more damaging to hair than the simple tinting process.

DAMAGE FROM BLEACHING

My hair is breaking off and becoming thin as a result of bleaching. Will this damage be permanent?

If hair is bleached excessively, it may become harsh and straw-like; extensive breaking is not uncommon. This damage occurs because peroxide, the bleaching agent, attacks keratin (the protein that is the principal constituent of hair, and of skin and nails) as well as hair-color pigment, causing the hair to lose its elasticity, resilience, and tensile strength. However, the damage is limited to that portion of the hair that is treated. Future hair growth is not affected, because the growing or living portion of the hair is located well below the scalp surface. Extensive breakage close to the scalp surface may be mistaken for hair loss; since hair growth averages one-half inch per month, it may take many months for hair to regrow to the desired length.

The extent of hair damage depends on several variables, one of which is the degree of bleaching. For instance, the high degree of bleaching necessary to make hair platinum blond may also make it dangerously brittle. Needless to say, when hair is damaged to this extent, bleaching should be discontinued to allow new hair to grow.

BLEACHING FOR EXTREME LIGHTENING

Just how difficult and how damaging to the hair is it to change the color from dark brown or black to pale blond?
This is one of the most complicated and potentially damaging of all color changes. Most or all of the original color must be "stripped out" by prebleaching to achieve the desired effect. Several applications of bleach may be required to remove existing color, and applications should be spaced several days apart. This may weaken the hair and make it harsh and straw-like, unless the bleaching is done properly. A toner is applied after stripping to give the hair the shade of color desired.

Because of the drastic color change, new hair growth is more conspicuous, so retouching is required more frequently. If bleaching is continued for a long time, the hair may become extremely dry and brittle, with a tendency to break off close to the scalp.

SUNLAMPS TO BLEACH HAIR

My hair is dark blond. I would like to make it lighter and brighter, but I don't want to use bleach. Would exposure to the sun or a sun lamp be a safe and effective means of bleaching it?
While heavy exposure to sunlight usually has a bleaching effect on hair, the intensity of radiation available from a sun-lamp is not sufficient to produce this effect. Moreover, bleaching produced by sunlight is not generally considered desirable since it produces a streaked, uneven effect and often leaves the hair dry and damaged.

If you wish to lighten and brighten your hair, you may want to try a "gentle lightener." This bleaching product provides just a mild lightening similar to the effect of sunlight on the hair. Such products produce little discomfort and minimal damage to hair. Sample brands are listed in the brand-name guide at the end of this chapter. You may also find that one of the permanent or semipermanent oxidation dyes will give satisfactory results. These products can lighten hair as much as two or three shades with relative safety.

FROSTING, TIPPING, PAINTING, AND STREAKING HAIR

I have heard the terms frosting, tipping, painting, and streaking used to describe the technique in which only portions of the hair are bleached. Are these terms synonymous? Will this procedure damage my hair or scalp?

Frosting, tipping, painting, and streaking all involve bleaching portions of the hair, but each technique gives a different effect. Frosting gives an overall salt-and-pepper effect to the hair by bleaching tiny strands throughout to blend with the darker hair. Tipping is identical to frosting, except that bleaching is confined to the tips of the hair. Streaking gives dramatic strips of lighter color around the face by bleaching one or more broad strands of hair. If bleach is applied with a paint brush to the outside of the hair, in either chosen or random patterns, the process is known as hair painting.

One of two methods may be used for frosting or tipping. In the first, a plastic cap is placed on the head; selected hairs are pulled through small holes in the cap and then bleached. In the second method, which takes longer, a few strands of hair are selected and placed on a small square of aluminum foil; bleach is applied starting half an inch from the scalp to the tip, or just to the tips, and the foil is wrapped around the hair until the bleaching process is completed. The procedure is repeated until the desired effect is achieved. The second method is also used for streaking. After bleaching, a toner may be applied for desirable shade.

Three advantages of these procedures compared with overall bleaching are: (1) the bleaching solution does not reach the scalp, (2) all of the hair is not involved, and (3) the procedures do not have to be repeated as frequently as all-over bleaching. The effect on the fibers that have been treated is the same as in the bleaching process. Frosting or bleaching aids in the manageability of fine hair because these processes add body to the hair. However, as discussed previously, any bleaching process also modifies the hair.

Since in frosting, tipping, painting, or streaking the bleaching solution does not reach the scalp, these methods may be more satisfactory to those for whom regular bleaching procedures result in scalp irritation.

TONERS

What kind of dye is a toner? Why is a toner needed when hair is bleached?
The mere bleaching of hair, to any depth desired, will sometimes produce an attractive shade in itself. Much more often, however, the shade noted after bleaching is raw, strawlike, or reddish. It usually is desirable to cover this shade with a light application of dye, both to neutralize the red tone and to create a more interesting color. The application of dye is the second step in a two-step process and is called "toning," the dyes being "toners."

The entire process of bleaching and toning is sometimes called a "double process." The dyes may be of the oxidation type, like the permanent tints, or they may be nonoxidation toners, which are similar to semipermanent dyes.

BRAND-NAME GUIDE TO HAIR COLORING PREPARATIONS

The following lists contain the most popular brands in each category alphabetically; no attempt is made to list all products in the category on the market:

Temporary Hair Colors

Come Alive Gray (Clairol)	Rinse
Fanci-Full Rinse (Roux)	Leave-in
Nestle Protein Colorinse (Nestlé-Le Mur)	Rinse
Noreen Color Hair Rinse (Noreen)	Rinse
Picture Perfect Instant Color Rinse (Clairol)	Rinse
Streaks 'n' Tips (Nestlé-Le Mur)	Leave-in

Semipermanent Hair Colors

Color 'n' Tone (Nestlé-Le Mur)	
Happiness (Clairol)	Aerosol
Loving Care Color Foam (Clairol)	Aerosol
Loving Care Hair Color Lotion (Clairol)	
Silk & Silver Hair Color Lotion (Clairol)	
Touch of Silver (L'Oréal)	

Vegetables Dyes

Egyptian Henna (Hopkins)

Metallic Dyes

Coffelt's Hair Color Restorer (Coffelt Chem. Co.)
Grecian Formula 16 (Combe)
Lady Grecian Formula (Combe)
RD for Men (Bishop Industries)
Youthair (Majestic Drug Co.)

Oxidation Tints

Breck Hair Color (Breck)	Shampoo-in
California Blonde (Max Factor)	Shampoo-in
Clairol Balsam Color (Clairol)	Shampoo-in
Colorsilk (Revlon)	Shampoo-in
European Naturals (Alberto-Culver)	Shampoo-in
Excellence Extra Rich Hair Color (L'Oréal)	Retouch
Excellence Permanent Shampoo-In Color (L'Oréal)	Shampoo-in

Fanci-Tone (Roux)	Retouch
For Brunettes Only (Alberto-Culver)	Shampoo-in
Look of Nature (Gillette)	Aerosol
Miss Clairol Hair Color Bath: Creme Formula (Clairol)	Retouch
Miss Clairol Natural Wear Shampoo Formula (Clairol)	Shampoo-in
New Dawn (Alberto-Culver)	Shampoo-in
New Dawn 2 (Alberto-Culver)	Shampoo-in
Nice 'n Easy (Clairol)	Shampoo-in
Preference (L'Oréal)	Shampoo-in
Tried and True (Max Factor)	Shampoo-in
True Brunette (Clairol)	Shampoo-in

Bleaches

Born Blonde Lightener (Clairol)	
Lady Clairol Whipped Creme Hair Lightener (Clairol)	
Lemon Go Lightly (Clairol)	Gentle lightener
Lite Creme Hair Lightener (Nestlé-Le Mur)	
L'Oréal Super Blonde (L'Oréal)	
L'Oréal Super Blue Creme Oil Lightener (L'Oréal)	
L'Oréal Young Blonde (L'Oréal)	Gentle lightener
Maxi-Blonde Lady Clairol (Clairol)	
Midnight Sun (Clairol)	Gentle lightener
Naturally Blonde Lightener (Clairol)	
Roux White Speed Bleach (Roux)	
Snowsilk Lightener (Revlon)	
Summer Blonde (Clairol)	
Sun-In (Gillette)	Gentle lightener
Ultra Blue Lady Clairol (Clairol)	
Ultrasilk Hair Lightener Kit (Revlon)	

Hair Toners

Blondsilk (Revlon)	Oxidation Type*

* Shampoo-in.

Born Blonde Lotion Toner (Clairol)	Nonoxidation type*
Clairol Creme Toner (Clairol)	Oxidation type†
Colorsilk Crystal-Lights Toner (Revlon)	Oxidation type* using crystals
L'Oréal Preference Perfect Blondes (L'Oréal)	Oxidation type*
Naturally Blonde (Clairol)	Oxidation type*

Frosting, Etc.

Frost & Tip (Clairol)

Hair Coloring for Men

Great Day, Regular and Concentrated (Clairol)	Semipermanent
See also Metallic Dyes	

Color Removers

Delete Color Remover (Roux)
Effasol (L'Oréal)
L'Oréal Hair Color Remover Kit (L'Oréal)
Metalex (Clairol)
Remov-Zit (Clairol)

* Shampoo-in.
† Retouch.

7

Hair Waving
and Straightening

HAIR-WAVING PROCEDURE

*How is hair waved in permanent waving? What ingredi-
ents are contained in permanent waving preparations?*
Most hair-waving preparations on the market today are ma-
chineless or cold-wave preparations. These were introduced
about the time of World War II and completely changed the
hair-waving industry. Formerly, permanent waving required
the application of heat, usually by a machine. Since cold-
wave preparations do not require outside heat, home-permanent waving became possible for the first time with their introduction.

The way hair is curled by cold wave preparations might
be compared to making Jell-O. Hair is chemically changed to
a flexible form like soft Jell-O, then shaped as desired and
allowed to set or harden for a "permanent" effect.

The essential ingredients in cold wave preparations are
most often chemicals known as thioglycolates. A waving lotion is applied that softens the hair, disrupting chemical
bonds within the hair protein. The hair then accepts a curled
position when it is wound around a curler or roller, or formed
into a pincurl, depending on the amount of curl, wave, or
"permanence" desired.

After a specified time (usually 10 to 20 minutes) the hair

must be rinsed with water and "neutralized," a step that locks the hair into the newly curled pattern. This usually involves the use of a separate solution containing an oxidizing agent such as hydrogen peroxide, which neutralizes the waving reaction quickly and completely. Some kits for home use allow for self-neutralization by air oxidation. This method is not widely used, however, since the hair must dry slowly on the curlers for at least six hours.

REACTIONS FROM PERMANENT WAVING

Does permanent waving damage hair or cause other reactions?

Reactions to permanent-wave solutions are comparatively rare, considering their extensive use. Complaints of hair damage due to cold waves were not infrequent, however, when such preparations were first introduced thirty years ago. Now a considerable amount of sound scientific information is available to guide the manufacturer in formulation of products that are safe under normal conditions of use. Solutions intended for home applications are usually weaker than those used in beauty salons, a precaution exercised by the manufacturer to reduce the possibility of hair damage in the event that the consumer ignores directions for use. Beauticians are assumed to have sufficient training and experience to handle stronger solutions without difficulty.

The most common complaints after permanent waving are brittleness, frizziness, split ends, and breakage close to the scalp. This damage ordinarily results from overprocessing. That is, the hair-waving solution is left on the hair too long or the hair is inadequately "neutralized." Other complaints include allergic reactions and burns on the scalp or skin.

If you plan to use a home preparation, be sure to carefully read and follow the directions for use. And don't assume that different brands can be used in the same manner. Finally, be sure your hair is in good condition before you begin; damaged or overbleached hair demands special attention if good results are to be achieved without further damage to the hair.

WAVING BLEACHED HAIR

My hair is bleached, and I'd like to get a permanent. Can I do this safely?

Bleaching is a chemical process that results in a permanent modification of the hair fiber. The tensile strength of the fiber is reduced and porosity increased. The amount of change depends on the original hair color and the amount of lightening that has been done. Very dark hair that is highly bleached will be more extensively altered than light hair bleached to the same shade. Bleached hair, therefore, can be relatively strong or weak.

If there is any question about the fragility of hair as a result of bleaching, one lock of hair should be tested with the permanent waving solution. A qualified beautician will recognize damaged hair when it exists and may be able to wave your hair properly even under these adverse conditions.

HAIR WAVING AND PREGNANCY

Is it true that permanent waving is not successful during pregnancy?

While some beauticians, on the basis of experience and observation, state that permanents are less successful at this time, we are not aware of any scientific evidence to support their opinion. In a normal, healthy woman, there should be no significant difference in the ability of the hair to curl during pregnancy.

This statement is readily supported by facts and simple arithmetic. All hair visible at the time pregnancy begins is nonviable (dead) hair and is not subject to physiologic alteration. This hair can be altered only by external treatments such as bleaches, waving preparations, or hair straighteners.

New hair grows at an average rate of one-half inch per month, or 4½ inches in 9 months. This new growth will be that portion of hair closest to the scalp and the hair least involved in the permanent-waving process. That part of the hair farthest from the scalp is older hair, which should respond to permanent waving in precisely the same manner it did prior to pregnancy.

Sometimes the degree of oiliness of hair changes during pregnancy, because the activity of oil glands of the scalp may be altered. This could affect the texture or feeling of the hair and its appearance, but changes in the degree of oiliness should not affect the action of permanent-waving preparations.

PERMANENT-WAVE FAILURE

Recently I had a permanent that didn't "take." My beautician blamed the failure on a tranquilizer I was taking at the time. Could this have been the cause?

We are skeptical of a connection between a drug taken internally and the action of permanent-wave lotions on the hair.

In the permanent-waving procedure an alkaline waving solution (usually containing thioglycolic acid) is applied. This solution, in the recommended concentration and properly applied, softens the hair and alters its chemical bonds so that the hair accepts a new waved configuration when it is wound around curlers or rollers. After the desired degree of waving is achieved, a neutralizer (an oxidizing agent) is applied. It sets the chemical bonds in the new curled configuration to produce a "permanent" waved effect.

Permanent waves fail for numerous reasons. Hair texture is one important factor. Fine, limp hair usually resists permanent waving and a fairly strong lotion is required. Hair that is wiry, brittle, or damaged resists waving and is subject to further damage, so special care is required to achieve a satisfactory wave. Some permanent-wave lotions must remain on the hair for a long time to alter the chemical bonds; if the wave solution is removed from the hair too soon, insufficient waving results. Beauticians sometimes do not thoroughly read and/or closely follow the manufacturer's directions for use—which may change as the product formulation (but not the trademark) is changed.

If the neutralizer is not applied, is not left on long enough, or does not work for some reason, the chemical bonds will revert to their previous form. Neutralizers that contain hydrogen peroxide will sometimes become inactivated before use. If this occurs, the neutralizer will be ineffective and the wave will not "take."

SAFETY OF ELECTRIC ROLLERS

Are electric hair rollers safe?
With newer electric hair setters, electricity is used only to heat the rollers. When you set your hair, these rollers are no longer connected to anything electrical, so there is no hazard from electric shock. Since the rollers must not be too hot to handle, they usually are not hot enough to damage hair. However, if used too frequently, they may cause your hair to become excessively dry and brittle. Other aspects of electric curlers are discussed in the following exchange.

ELECTRIC ROLLERS AND HAIR DAMAGE

Do electrically heated rollers for "quick sets" damage hair?
Electric hair rollers are usually made of heavy plastic and come in sets of approximately twenty. In most units rollers are electrically heated on upright rods or mandrels, all of which are enclosed in a plastic container. Electric curling units have automatic cutoff switches designed to turn off the heating element when the rollers have reached a certain temperature. Some have a thermal safety fuse as well. Reports have been

received that some units without fuses don't always cut off, thus increasing the danger of burns from touching the hot rollers.

More recently, steam-heated rollers have become popular. Rollers heated on rods may become hotter than steam-heated rollers and therefore produce longer-lasting curls, but in case of equipment failure they may have greater potential for burning the hair or scalp.

If electric rollers are used too frequently, they may have a drying effect on the hair; they should not be used daily.

A tighter, longer lasting set will be obtained from the usual wash, set, dry procedure. Electric rollers are best used for touch-up sets between shampoos.

CURLING IRONS

Can you advise me about the safety of electric hair-curling irons? I've always wanted to try this method of curling because it's so much quicker than the wet, set, dry method.

Electric hair-curling devices for home use work on the same principle as old-fashioned curling irons. Whereas the old-fashioned irons required heating in a flame, newer devices are heated by an electric current. With either device, the hair is curled by heat emanating from the curling iron.

If the heat is too low, your hair will not be curled adequately. If the heat is too high, your hair will be damaged, become fragile and dry. Generally, if the curling iron is hot enough to burn your fingers it will also burn your hair.

The heat generated by most electric curling irons is low enough to be relatively safe. However, the results will probably not be as satisfactory or as long-lasting as advertising claims lead you to believe. A curling iron may serve some purpose as a supplement, when there is no time for the regular wet, set, dry method, but it cannot replace it.

Curling irons are plugged in when you use them on your hair, but are electrically safe if you follow the manufacturer's directions with special care. Curling irons are much hotter than electric curlers; hair and scalp damage can result from careless or excessive use.

WAVE-SETTING PREPARATIONS

A variety of wave-setting preparations are available today— gels, liquids in squirt bottles, aerosol sprays, aerosol foams, and old-fashioned liquids. How do these products differ? How can I tell which one is best for my hair?

Wave-setting preparations have been undergoing rapid changes in recent years. For many years these products were semiliquid gels based on natural gums. Modern wave-setting preparations contain various synthetic polymers instead of gums and come in a variety of forms.

Gum-based wave sets, a few of which are still available today, have many deficiencies. They are clumsy to apply, lack uniformity and flexibility, flake badly on the hair, reduce glossiness, and are subject to bacterial contamination. Modern preparations have overcome most of these deficiencies. Present ingredients vary according to brand and form (i.e., gel, liquid, or aerosol), but any of these products should provide satisfactory sets when used according to the manufacturer's directions. The amount of wave set will determine to a large extent the softness or firmness of the set. Too little set, such as one quick spray from an aerosol, will do little or nothing. Too much wave set will make the hair dull and result in flaking that may resemble dandruff. Most manufacturers provide different formulations for hard-to-set hair and normal hair. Some incorporate extra ingredients to condition hair, provide antistatic action, or add sheen or luster.

The only way you can determine which type you will prefer is to try various products. The method of application may be the deciding point. For instance, you dip your fingers into a gel and apply it to your hair; you pour a liquid into your palm, rub your hands together, and work it into your hair; and you spray an aerosol foam, an aerosol spray, or a liquid in a squirt bottle directly onto your hair and comb it through before setting. A liquid in a squirt bottle or an aerosol can also be sprayed directly on rollers or pincurls after setting.

EFFECT OF CURL-HOLDER SPRAYS ON HAIR COLOR

After a "curl-holder" preparation was sprayed on my hair, the hair developed an orange color. What could have caused this reaction? What can I do to regain my original hair color?

Many "curl-holder" preparations contain shellac, which helps to stiffen hair. If such a preparation is applied to dyed hair, there occasionally is a reaction between the shellac or alcohol solvent and the existing hair dye. The result of this reaction is discolored hair.

It is also possible that corrosion occurred in the curl-holder aerosol container. If so, when the product was used a rust-colored deposit was applied to your hair.

Undesired color from either of these causes usually can be removed by shampooing with your regular shampoo, to which some ethyl alcohol has been added. This will help to dissolve and wash away the shellac and the color without injuring your hair.

SETTING FINE HAIR

How can I give my fine hair enough body so that it will hold a set?

Naturally fine hair cannot be changed permanently since it is an inherited characteristic. But certain cosmetic measures can give fine hair more body to help it hold a set.

A medium-short, blunt-cut style is one way to add body to fine hair. A professional or home-permanent wave is another method. If you don't want a great deal of curl, use a body-wave kit designed especially for hair that is difficult to set.

A setting gel will also help your hair hold a set. Be generous when you apply the gel. Use more of it on the parts of your hair that are most resistant to curl.

PSORIASIS AND PERMANENT WAVING

I have a mild case of psoriasis of the scalp. Would it be safe to have a permanent?

This is a medical decision that should be made by the physician who is treating your psoriasis and is familiar with your particular case. In some cases, permanent waving or other hair treatments are allowed; in other cases, such procedures may aggravate the condition.

Most people who have psoriasis should be under the care of a physician. Although psoriasis has no known cure, various medications and treatments are available to improve the condition. The person who has self-diagnosed the condition as psoriasis may have something else and would benefit from a medical consultation. (See the discussion of psoriasis in Chapter 21, "Other Skin Problems.")

HAIR-STRAIGHTENING METHODS

What methods are available for hair straightening?

Three methods are used to straighten naturally curly hair: (1) application of pomades or resinous fixatives, (2) passing a heated comb through the hair (hot pressing), and (3) the use of chemical straighteners. Until recent years, only the use of pomade was practiced for straightening hair in homes, because hot pressing and chemical straightening procedures were sufficiently complicated and/or hazardous that they were conducted primarily in beauty shops. During the late sixties, however, newer chemical straighteners were introduced for home use. A discussion of each type follows.

HAIR POMADES

How safe and effective are pomades for straightening hair? The use of pomades (heavy oils or petrolatum-type products) was probably the earliest means of controlling extremely curly hair. These products plaster the hair against the scalp and remove some of the curliness by strictly mechanical means; no chemical changes in the hair are involved. The straightening results are temporary. Because they result in greasiness, pomades are not used extensively by women. They are more effective on short hair and are used mainly by men.

Pomades occasionally produce a contact dermatitis in people who may be sensitive (allergic) to the perfume or other ingredients in the products. They also may cause outbreaks of skin blemishes along the hairline.

HEAT METHOD FOR HAIR STRAIGHTENING

How is hair straightened by the "hot pressing" method? Are there any dangers?
Hot pressing or combing to straighten hair was introduced in 1910 and has been widely practiced, primarily in beauty shops. After shampooing and towel drying, a small amount of pressing oil is distributed through the hair. The oil serves as a heat-transfer medium and as a lubricant for hot combing. A metal pressing comb, heated to 300° to 500° F., is passed quickly through a tress of hair. The high temperature breaks some of the intermolecular bonds within the hair and permits it to straighten under the tension of the hot combing. The hair temperature drops rapidly as the comb passes through, the broken bonds unite in their new position, and the hair retains its new straightened position, but only temporarily.

Exposure of hot combed hair to water, high humidity, or even to scalp perspiration causes it to revert to its original curly configuration.

First- to third-degree burns are the most common skin damage that results from hot pressing of the hair. Faulty technique, carelessness, and repeated use of the hot comb can cause substantial hair damage. When hair is burned, the resulting patches of broken hair will give the appearance of partial baldness. Hair almost always regrows satisfactorily if repeated heat treatments are avoided. (Heat damage to hair is discussed further in Chapter 12, "Other Hair Problems.")

IRONING TO STRAIGHTEN HAIR

My teenaged daughter has been ironing her hair to make it straight enough for a long, straight look. Will this damage her hair?

The teenage practice of ironing hair is not recommended. Heat can damage hair temporarily, making it fragile and dry, with subsequent breakage. Also, the scalp can be burned accidentally. If your daughter wants to have her hair straightened, we would recommend that she use one of the chemical preparations designed specifically for this purpose.

CHEMICAL HAIR STRAIGHTENERS

What do chemical hair-straightening products contain? Are any hazards associated with their use?

Three types of chemical hair straighteners are now available: (1) alkaline (sodium hydroxide) creams, (2) thioglycolate lotions or creams, and (3) ammonium or sodium bisulfite lotions. These hair straighteners react with and alter the chemical structure of hair to provide generally permanent uncurling. In other words, the hair does not revert to its original curly state on exposure to water, shampooing, or high humidity. A discussion of each type of chemical hair straightener follows. A brand-name guide to these products, by type, appears at the end of the chapter.

ALKALI STRAIGHTENERS

Are alkali hair straighteners hazardous to use?
These straighteners contain strongly caustic ingredients. They act by swelling the hair and breaking and altering chemical bonds in the hair fibers.

This action is very rapid and the fibers relax quickly under tension of combing. The hair is then rinsed with water to stop the chemical action. Because of their rapid chemical action, these products must be left on the hair no longer than 5 to 10 minutes; otherwise the hair may be seriously damaged. To minimize the possibility of first- to third-degree chemical burns, the scalp and skin are usually covered with a protective cream. Marked contact dermatitis with swelling of the face and scalp has been reported from exposure to alkali curl relaxers, especially where a protective cream has not been used or proper care has not been exercised during the curl-removal process.

The greatest potential hazard of alkali straighteners is direct contact with the eyes, which can cause immediate and possibly permanent damage. Fortunately, these products are usually provided in very thick lotion or cream form, and accidental contamination of the eyes is rare. For safety reasons, alkali curl relaxers are limited primarily to beauty shop usage.

THIOGLYCOLATE STRAIGHTENERS

How do thioglycolate straighteners compare with other chemical straighteners?
Thioglycolate straighteners, whose active ingredients are also present in permanent-waving lotions, have been in limited

use for curl relaxing for several years. They are used for "reverse" waving to remove curl from hair rather than to curl it. Thioglycolate straightening is most often done in beauty salons, although a few products are available for home use.

Thioglycolate lotions are applied to and allowed to remain on clean, damp hair for 10 to 15 minutes. The hair is combed for 10 to 20 minutes. Thioglycolates break some of the chemical bonds of the hair. It is then rinsed with water and neutralized with an oxidative solution, which rebuilds new bonds to produce hair that is straight instead of curly.

Unfortunately, thioglycolate straighteners are not normally as effective as desired. They cause relatively little damage to hair and scalp when used as directed, although straightening hair already damaged by earlier chemical treatments such as bleaching or dyeing should be avoided to prevent breakage. Occasional mild scalp irritations that clear up within a few days have been reported.

BISULFITE STRAIGHTENERS

How safe and effective are bisulfite straighteners?
Bisulfite straighteners are the most recent development in the chemical hair-straightening field. Products are available for both professional and home use. (The term "curl relaxer" instead of "straightener" is commonly used to describe them.) Bisulfite curl relaxers are more extensively used for straightening hair in the home than any other type of chemical straightener.

Like thioglycolates, they produce reversible changes of certain chemical bonds in the hair. Bisulfite lotion is applied to clean, damp hair, which is then covered with a plastic turban for about 15 minutes. Next the hair is combed for 15 to 20 minutes to produce the degree of straightening desired. The hair's chemical bonds are then relinked in their new orientation by rinsing the hair with water and then with an alkaline stabilizer solution. A conditioner is applied to the hair as the final step.

The effectiveness of bisulfite relaxers is similar to that of hot combing, but is more permanent. The result is also equivalent to that of caustic alkali straighteners and superior to the thioglycolate method.

CHEMICAL STRAIGHTENERS: LIMITATIONS AND PRECAUTIONS

How effective are chemical straighteners on very curly hair? What special precautions should be observed in their use?

With present technology, there is no satisfactory way to go safely from extremely curly or kinky hair to completely straight hair with any of the chemical straighteners. Some degree of straightening can be obtained, but users must be realistic in their expectations.

Bisulfite curl relaxers are mild on the scalp and skin, and chances of hair damage appear considerably less than from other types of chemical hair straightening products. As with all chemical treatments, however, the manufacturer's directions and precautions should be carefully observed. If hair is dry, brittle, or damaged or tends to break easily, a curl relaxer should not be used. If the hair has been bleached, color-treated, or previously straightened by other methods, a curl relaxer should be used with caution. A test should be performed on a small section before the product is applied to all of the hair. Manufacturers include directions for applying this test (a strand test) and for interpreting the results. A curl relaxer should not be used if the scalp or skin is sensitive, scaly, scratched, sore, or tender.

Directions and precautions should be reviewed and followed carefully every time a product is used—not just the first time. Unsatisfactory and harmful effects frequently result from not following directions.

HAIR STRAIGHTENING VS. WAVING

I understand that hair straightening and hair waving preparations contain the same ingredients. Are the hazards comparable?

Not all hair-straightening products contain thioglycolates, the ingredients commonly used in hair waving preparations (see preceding answers). Even when the same principal ingredients are used, their concentrations and the nature and amounts of other components in the preparations differ significantly. However, when straightening is done with a product that does contain thioglycolate, the potential for scalp irritation and damage may be greater than with permanent waving. In permanent waving, the waving lotion is usually applied after the hair has been wrapped in curlers. Thus the application can be controlled so that little of the chemical comes in contact with the scalp. When the same material is used for straightening, it is applied to hair all over the scalp, thus increasing the chances of scalp irritation.

STRAIGHTENING BLEACHED HAIR

Is it safe to have dyed or bleached hair straightened?

We understand that some manufacturers of hair-straightening products supply one type of product for normal hair and another for dyed or bleached hair. Since dyed or, particularly, bleached hair may already be altered from its normal state by the coloring processes, great care should be taken and a specially formulated product should be used to avoid excessive breakage. From the safety viewpoint it is advisable to forego straightening until new, unbleached hair has grown out. Hair damage that can result from bleaching is discussed in the previous chapter.

BRAND-NAME GUIDE TO CHEMICAL
HAIR-STRAIGHTENING PRODUCTS*

Sulfite-Bisulfite Products

Charles Antell Curl Relaxing Formula—Charles Antell
Curlaxer—Curlaxer Corp. (Posner)
Curl Free—Prom Cosmetics/Gillette Company
U.N.C.U.R.L.—Clairol
Vege-Kurl—Vege-Kurl, Inc.

Thioglycolate Products

Allyn's Professional Hair Straightening Cream—Continental Beauty
    Supply, Inc.
Curl-Away—Continental Laboratories, Inc.
Curl Out for Fine or Normal Hair—Posner
Curl Out for Tinted and Bleached Hair—Posner
Curls Away—Richard Hudnut
Go Straight—Nutritonic
Less Curl Creme Hair Straightener—House of Lontay
Lontay Creme Hair Straightener—House of Lontay
Perma Silk—Daggett & Ramsdell
Perma Strate—Perma Strate Co.
Royal Crown Hair Relaxer for Medium and Fine Hair—J. Strickland
    & Co.
Set Me Straight—Rexall
Silky Strate—Living Beauty, Inc.
Smooth Away—Helene Curtis
Smooth 'N Straight—Gabrieleen
Straight Set—Max Factor
Sudden Silk—Evans Chemetics Co.
Wellastrate—Wella

Sodium Hydroxide (Alkali) Products

Apex Natural Perm—Apex Beauty Products
Curl Out for Coarse and Extra Curly Hair—Posner
Curl Out for Professional Use—Posner
Ever Perm—Helene Curtis
Hair Strate—Summit Laboratories
Mr. Fredericks—Gran-Gay
Pastel Princess Permanent—Summit Laboratories
Royal Crown Relaxer Permanent for Coarse Hair—J. Strickland & Co.
Ultra Sheen—Johnson Products Co.
Ultra Wave—Johnson Products Co.

*This list is based on information available to us at publication time. Manufacturers may change the composition and/or ingredients of a product without changing the brand name. The products listed have not been evaluated for safety and effectiveness; no endorsement is intended or permitted. This list includes samples of each type of chemical hair straightener; it does not attempt to include all brand names. Some of these products have limited distribution.

DAMAGE TO LONG HAIR FROM STRAIGHTENING

*I have been straightening my long, curly hair, and now it
is breaking off. Can you recommend a treatment to stop
the breakage?*

The first thing you should know is that long hair is old hair.
Since hair grows about 6 inches per year, the ends of long
hair may be 2 years old. For 2 years this part of the hair has
been subjected to various chemical and physical stresses, so
it isn't surprising that the ends tend to split and/or to break
off.

Damaged hair cannot be restored to its previous normal
state. It would be best to cut off the part of your hair that is
damaged and allow new, undamaged hair to grow out. Further
physical and chemical injury to your hair should be minimized
to the greatest extent possible. Don't bleach, dye, or straighten
your hair until new, undamaged hair has grown out. Damaged
hair may undergo more extensive, unpredictable damage from
some of these processes than does normal hair.

Combing and brushing should be limited to what is
necessary for good grooming and should be gently performed.
The mechanical force necessary to comb the ends of long hair
is far greater than that required to comb the ends of short
hair, and increased mechanical force contributes to hair
breakage.

After shampooing, pat your hair dry—don't rub it. Apply
a postshampoo conditioner to help minimize tangling and
restore sheen to damaged hair. Use a wide-toothed comb to
gently comb wet hair; don't brush it, as this may increase
breakage. And avoid overexposing your hair to summer sun,
which increases dryness.

Periodic oil treatments before shampoos may also be
helpful. (See exchange on hot oil treatments for hair.)

8

Miscellaneous
Hair Products

SHOPPING FOR THE RIGHT SHAMPOO

What's the latest word on shampoo? So many different kinds are being sold. Do extra ingredients such as egg, herbs, beer, and protein really help your hair?

A shampoo is basically water, detergent, and usually some fatty material. The main ingredient is the detergent. This loosens dirt and grease (oil) and cleans your hair. The most important thing a consumer should know is how much detergent a particular shampoo contains—and this varies considerably. A recent British survey of eighty-two different shampoos, many of them the same as those sold in the United States, revealed a range of detergent concentrations from less than 5 to more than 20 percent. Some shampoos for oily hair, for example, had more detergent than those of the same brand for dry hair—but about as many didn't (although they did tend to have less fatty material or none at all).

Unfortunately, you have no way of knowing how much detergent a particular shampoo contains. Your only course is trial and error. You might find, for example, that you need two or three times more of one shampoo than another to get your hair clean. But don't assume that because a shampoo is thick it's concentrated. Manufacturers can thicken shampoos without making them stronger.

The study also showed that no specially formulated shampoo gave any added benefits consistently. Detergent loosens dirt and oil, and all three are washed away in the rinse. Any other ingredients in the shampoo also end up down the drain. Specifically, the study led to the following conclusions about some of the more popular added ingredients:

Lemon oil does not cut grease any better than detergent alone—and neither does lime oil. A lemon rinse helps only if hair is washed with soap and hard water; it eliminates the soap "scum"—but most modern shampoos have a detergent base and don't leave any residue.

Beer makes hair easier to set if used in the final rinse. Mixed in and rinsed off with shampoo, it does nothing.

Egg or egg yolk, used with warm water, is an effective "shampoo" for hair that is not very dirty. But the solution is rinsed out and provides no additional benefits. As an added ingredient, egg provides no special bonus.

Herb shampoos, promoted for both normal hair and problem hair, possess characteristic odors but otherwise provide no special benefits.

Although some protein shampoos, such as egg and beer shampoos, have been in use for many years, the present use of the term *protein* shampoo is really a misnomer. Many shampoo products are said to contain protein, but they don't. They are made instead with compounds derived from protein. The principal selling claim for these shampoos is that they mend or help to mend split ends. However, actual use tests do not support this. In one experiment, a group of people with split ends tested the effects of a "protein" shampoo against a regular shampoo. At the end of 2 months, 20 percent of those using the protein product reported that they had fewer split ends—but so did 20 percent of those using the ordinary shampoo. Furthermore, a laboratory test involving repeated washings of split end hairs from girls' heads showed no significant differences between "protein" and ordinary shampoos.

The British study concluded:

> Shampoos and hair vary. So it's quite likely that one shampoo may deal better with one head of hair than another shampoo. As it is impossible to know in advance what is going to suit you, it makes sense to start off with a small size of an inexpensive or popular brand and experiment until you find the product that best suits your hair. And don't be persuaded into feeding your hair things it can't digest—especially protein.

INEXPENSIVE SHAMPOOS

> *My five children insist on shampooing their hair three and four times a week to get the "dry, natural" look. I say they're ruining their hair, they say no. If they wash their hair this frequently, can they safely use the off-brand bargain shampoos sold in discount drugstores and supermarkets?*

Your kids are right. Most adolescents have excessively oily hair and frequent, even daily, shampooing is needed to control the oiliness.

It's difficult to make a blanket statement about off-brand shampoos. Some may be diluted and, while you're paying less than for a brand name product, you may be using more. Some may not contain conditioners, so you'll have to supplement the shampoo with a creme rinse or other conditioner. On the other hand, people with very fine and long hair often use a conditioner regardless of the type of shampoo they use.

Inexpensive products made by small manufacturers may not be adequately tested for such things as eye irritation potential (all shampoos have some irritation potential). Others, however, are "private labels" produced by large, brand-name manufacturers. In this case the product is the same as that sold in the expensive package.

Some inexpensive shampoos simply don't smell as good

as the expensive products. Most are not advertised, so you're not contributing to the manufacturer's advertising budget. And many are packaged less attractively and less expensively than "name" shampoos.

WATERLESS SHAMPOOS

My mother is an invalid and cannot have her hair shampooed frequently. Do you have any suggestions for keeping her hair well-groomed?

You might try supplementing regular shampooing with the use of a waterless or dry shampoo. These products most often consist of absorbent powder and a mild alkali. They are available as dry powders, aerosol foams or waterless liquids. Dry shampoos have been greatly improved in recent years; they are easier to apply and give better results than previously available products.

While waterless shampoos don't clean hair as thoroughly as do wet shampoos, they remove some surface oils, dirt, and odors, and are useful when illness or lack of time preclude regular shampooing.

The method of applying waterless shampoos varies according to the product, but the principle is the same. The product is applied to the hair, left for a few minutes, then brushed or toweled away. For best results, follow package directions.

SOAP VS. DETERGENT SHAMPOOS

How can I distinguish between soap and synthetic detergent shampoos?

This is a difficult task for the consumer because no standard statements appear on product labels. Some soap shampoo labels refer to soap "fats" such as coconut oil, olive oil, and palm oil. A detergent shampoo may be identified as such, or may be called "soapless." If the label doesn't have an identifying statement, you can assume that the product is a synthetic detergent or a mixture of detergent and soap. The trend in shampoos in recent years has been toward detergent-based products.

The selection of a detergent or soap shampoo depends on personal preference (unless you have a hair or scalp problem for which your physician has prescribed a specific product). Remember that properties of skin and hair, such as texture and degree of oiliness, are determined primarily by heredity.

In selecting a shampoo consider the following criteria:

1. The shampoo should cleanse hair and scalp thoroughly with one application unless your hair is quite oily.

2. Hair should be left soft, shining, and manageable.

3. The shampoo must rinse off easily and not leave any residue that might interfere with subsequent hair treatments.

4. It must not be irritating.

5. It must satisfy your tastes in color, perfume, texture, and lather.

6. It must be simple to apply.

RAINWATER AND ACID RINSES FOR SHAMPOOING

What are the benefits of using rainwater to shampoo hair? Is vinegar or lemon juice recommended as a rinse after shampooing?

Rainwater is "soft water" in the sense that it contains no extraneous minerals or salts. These substances, present in ordinary tap water to a greater or lesser extent, determine the so-called hardness of water. They react chemically with ordinary soap to form an insoluble "scum." The chemical action of a weak acid such as vinegar or lemon juice rinses the scum away. Since soap scum can make hair appear dull and lusterless, using a lemon juice rinse will leave it looking brighter.

An acid is not necessary if shampoo is used, since detergent shampoos do not leave deposits on hair.

CREME RINSES AND HAIR CONTROL

What are the benefits of using creme rinses on hair?
Shampooing decreases the hair's oily film, resulting in a dry and dull appearance. Static charges that make hair "fly" usually develop after it has been shampooed. This causes the hair to tangle easily, and combing may result in breakage.

Creme rinses are intended to help control these problems. They usually contain as a basic ingredient an antistatic compound that forms a residual film on the hair, giving it a soft feeling and improving its gloss. These preparations are especially beneficial for hair damaged by excessive bleaching, permanent waving or dyeing.

Claims that creme rinses will do more than make hair manageable are highly questionable.

BEER RINSES FOR HAIR

I have been using a beer rinse on my hair that seems to give it more "body" than anything I have used previously. What ingredients does beer contain that would produce this effect? Is beer more effective diluted or undiluted?
Some people insist that beer rinses are helpful for their hair, although there is no sound scientific evidence for this claim. The extra "body" that beer rinses might give to hair is probably due to two ingredients, sugar and protein-containing material. These probably cling to the hair and may appear to provide increased "body and manageability." Egg shampoos and creme rinses are used for much the same reason.

It has been said that beer gives hair a coarser feel. For some people it apparently is more effective undiluted. Others feel that undiluted beer makes their hair feel too coarse. Either way, the beer aroma is often left on the hair and may be considered undesirable.

Evidently, no one has ever evaluated the benefits of light

beer versus dark beer—although people with more expensive tastes have used champagne to seek the same results.

PROTEIN CONDITIONERS

Are protein conditioners really better for your hair? Does the protein in the conditioner get inside your hair and make it healthier?

Protein conditioners do not change hair structure, affect hair growth, or in any way permanently alter the hair. While hair does consist primarily of a type of protein known as keratin, the hair that is visible above the skin surface is dead tissue that cannot be revitalized. Furthermore, the protein derivatives incorporated into hair preparations are derived from animal tissue, not from human hair.

Protein conditioners have the same effect as other conditioners—they add "body" to thin hair and improve appearance and manageability, especially of damaged hair. They also help to minimize tangling and add gloss or luster. They coat the hair shaft with a film that is claimed to make thin hairs appear thicker. If the hair has been damaged—i.e., the outer layer has been chipped or cracked by teasing or bleaching—it is claimed that the conditioner smoothes and fills in the roughened, uneven surfaces in much the same way that a wood filler smoothes out cracks or scratches in wood furniture. Such patching, however, does nothing to strengthen the hair or restore its structure and, like all patching, is of a temporary nature.

LEMON GELATIN FOR HAIR RINSE

I've read that lemon-flavored gelatin makes an excellent wave-setting preparation. What is your opinion? Is it harmful?

Gelatin probably could be used as a rinse and wave-setting preparation, but we doubt that the results would be as satisfactory as those achieved from using a cosmetic preparation formulated for this purpose. Sugar and protein ingredients in the gelatin product may cling to the hair, giving an impression of increased manageability and body. The gelatin may help hair sets last longer in a way similar to regular wave-setting gels or lotions, but unless the right dilutions are used the gelatin may be too stiff.

It probably doesn't matter what flavor gelatin is used. Lemon-flavored gelatin may have been suggested because lemon juice is sometimes recommended as a rinse following shampoos and because lemon has a "fresh" aroma. Gelatin would not be harmful to hair, but the hair may appear dull and feel coarse if too much gelatin remains on it.

HAIR SPRAY AND LUNG DAMAGE

Can the use of hair sprays cause lung damage?
A number of reports indicate that physicians have seen various lung conditions in people exposed to long-term use of hair sprays. In particular, it has been alleged that thesaurosis—the accumulation of unusual amounts of normal or foreign substances in the body (here, the lungs)—has resulted from the use of hair sprays. In only a few reports calling attention to this claimed relationship has there been any attempt to provide more than circumstantial evidence, and to our knowledge the relationship and its effects have not been definitely established.

Experiments sponsored by the Food and Drug Administration involving laboratory animals failed to reveal any relationship between the use of hair sprays and lung damage. Industrial laboratories have also reported on carefully conducted experiments that appear to indicate that hair sprays do not constitute a health hazard. Studies involving hairdressers, who are exposed to hair sprays in their normal occupation, indicate little evidence to substantiate a link between the sprays and thesaurosis.

Most of us are familiar with the perfumed environment

produced when hair sprays are used. While the odor and fine mist persist for some time, larger and heavier particles containing most of the hair spray resin settle quickly. It's a good idea to use hair sprays in a large, well-ventilated area—but for reasons of comfort rather than health.

MEN'S HAIR-GROOMING PREPARATIONS

Can you recommend a men's hair lotion or cream that makes hair smoother and less coarse?

Many brands of men's hair grooming and conditioning products are available to help hold hair in place, make it feel smoother, impart sheen, and condition the scalp. However, they cannot affect the growth of hair or its texture; these are predetermined characteristics.

In the past, many hair-grooming aids for men were called "tonics," implying some therapeutic effect—although they usually contained no effective drugs or medications and did nothing more than groom the hair. This term is seldom used today.

Hair grooms and conditioners for men can be grouped as follows: (1) liquid and solid brilliantines and pomades, (2) alcoholic lotions, (3) emulsions, (4) clear gels, and (5) aerosols.

Brilliantines and Pomades: These products impart a high degree of sheen and lubricity. Solid or semisolid preparations have greater "grooming" qualities than liquids. Such products have been on the market since before the turn of the century, but modern forms are cosmetically more elegant and easier to use.

Alcoholic lotions: These are very popular. They are essentially oils in solutions with alcohol, most often a clear solution. The alcohol evaporates upon application to hair, leaving an oily film that acts as a light grooming aid. For many years castor oil was used extensively, but it has lost its popularity to synthetic oils that do not become rancid or discolored as do castor oil products. Alcoholic hair lotions are less greasy than brilliantines or pomades.

Emulsions: Emulsions and cream hair dressings were introduced during World War II, when alcohol for lotions became unavailable to the cosmetics industry. Emulsions in liquid and semisolid forms quickly became popular and dominated the market until recently. They are available in two basic types: oil-in-water emulsions and water-in-oil emulsions. The basic difference is that the former can be diluted with water and is readily rinsed from hands or hair. The latter is not dispersed in water and must be removed by soap or shampoo.

Creams, whether liquid or semisolid, are easy and pleasant to use, without the oily or greasy feeling of many brilliantines and pomades.

Mineral oil is still the basic ingredient in most of these emulsions but is combined with many other ingredients.

Clear gels: Clear gel hair dressings are a recent development. These are for the most part transparent gels, with all the desirable attributes of a good hair dressing plus a high degree of esthetic appeal. They consist of delicately balanced transparent compounds, actually oil-in-water emulsions. The oil, which may be mineral or vegetable, is dispersed as submicroscopic particles. Gels also contain water and may contain other ingredients.

A modification of clear gel is water-based gel with a low solids content. Gels of this type consist primarily of a high molecular weight, water-soluble synthetic polymer, with additives to plasticize and modify the film that remains on the hair. After the water evaporates, the hair is left with a light, flexible, transparent coating. These gels are greaseless and have excellent hair-grooming qualities with particular appeal to men. They are usually crystal clear, with small bubbles suspended throughout.

Aerosols: The latest development in men's hair-grooming products is the aerosol preparation. Two types of aerosols are available. One is basically a grooming aid similar to a brilliantine, but in aerosol form. The other is a modified hair spray. It differs from hair sprays marketed for women in that it deposits a softer film on the hair, does not produce a stiff crust, and has a more "masculine" fragrance or no fragrance at all. The chief advantage of aerosol preparations is convenience of use.

You may have to experiment with several different brands and types of products before you find the one most suited to your needs.

HAIR THICKENERS

I've been reading about new creams to put on hair after washing it that are supposed to make it thicker. How do these work? Are they likely to damage my hair in any way?
Creams that claim to "thicken" and add body to hair are similar to preparations that claim to treat damaged hair. They contain oils and proteins that coat the hair with an invisible film that does make it slightly thicker, thus giving it more body. These products also make hair feel smoother and make it more manageable. They are especially helpful if your hair is damaged.

These products won't damage your hair, but they won't change it either (the texture of hair cannot be changed). They coat hair to make it appear healthier, and this is fine, but for best results they must be applied after every shampoo.

HAND-HELD HAIR DRIERS

I've been thinking about buying a hand-held blower hair drier. What are the differences in results between these and hooded driers?
Hand-held blower driers are better for presently favored natural hair styles because hair can be shaped with the drier comb

attachments as it dries. In addition, hand-held driers work faster because their hot air can be more easily concentrated on specific areas of wet hair.

Some hand-held driers seem to blow very hot air. Are these acceptable for use?

If you plan to purchase a hand-held blower drier, look for the Underwriters Laboratories (UL) approval label on the drier. Underwriters Laboratories tests assure not only electrical safety in design, but also that the air temperature at the drier's nozzle is no more than 85°C. (153°F.) above room temperature and that the drier is equipped with a thermostat to shut it off in case it overheats for any reason. On the average, hand-held driers operate at somewhat higher temperatures than do hooded driers to achieve drying and styling effects in a short time. However, the hair being dried need not become overheated because the hand-held drier is moved over the hair (unlike the hooded drier), and thus never concentrates heat on any one spot for too long a time.

Still, can heat damage hair?

Without simultaneous manipulation, significant irreversible heat damage to hair occurs only above 150°C. (300°F.). (See the exchange on heat damage to hair in Chapter 12, "Other Hair Problems.")

Concerning potential damage to hair, remember that hair is subject to some physical damage (deterioration, weakening, breakage) from such commonplace manipulations as brushing and combing, towel drying, massage, washing, etc. Good hair care requires gentle handling of hair at all times. This applies even more strongly when hair is being dried. Any elevation in temperature softens hair and makes it more plastic and weaker. Damage to hair from the use of hand-held driers may, therefore, result not so much from excess temperatures—especially when the drier is of good quality—as from improper and overenthusiastic manipulation of hair while it is hot.

But if I want to style my hair with hand-held drier comb-and-brush attachments, I have to manipulate it.

The ability of hand-held driers to style hair relies on the easy plastic deformability of hair when it is hot, or when it is hot and wet. In itself, the plastic deformation does not harm hair. But the brush-and-comb attachments should be used with gentle, slow, and constant pulling—not rapid, jerky, high force strokes. The results will be better without prolonging drying time or damaging your hair.

Can these driers "overdry" hair, making it harsh and brittle?

Hair holds water within the fibers in a reversible way. The amount of water held in the fibers is 33 percent when hair is wet, zero in absolutely dry air at room temperature, and 13 percent at 65 percent relative humidity and 70°F. Even if hair is "overdried," it will pick up from the air within an hour the amount of water that corresponds to its surroundings. On the other hand, hair that is not dried completely will lose its water content in excess of that in the surrounding air. The hair condition that popularly is called "harsh and brittle" is not due to a deficiency in water content of the hair. At any rate, it is easier to avoid "overdrying" hair, even in spots, with hand-held driers than with hooded driers because the user can continuously feel the condition of the hair.

Are there any rules concerning safe use that are specific for hand-held driers?

Apart from the general rule valid for all electrical appliances—never use them in the tub or shower—there may be one that is somewhat specific for hand-held driers. *The air intake opening should never be covered when the drier is in operation.* If you cannot conveniently hold the drier during use without covering the air intake grill, even partially, select another type of drier. In addition, do not put the drier down without switching it off. Table surfaces or other objects may restrict the air intake in that position. In these cases, the drier may overheat somewhat before the thermostat shuts it off.

In conclusion, be sure to use a hair drier with a UL seal.

The styling manipulation of hot hair should be gentle with the hand-held drier. Do not use it in or under water, and do not cover the air intake while the drier is working.

HAIR ROLLERS AND CLIPS

Do brush rollers cause hair breakage any more than other rollers? Does it matter whether I use bobby pins, plastic pins, or metal clips to hold the rollers in place?

Any type of hair roller may cause a temporary hair loss (known as traction alopecia) if the rollers pull your hair too tightly. To avoid such pulling, wind your hair tightly around the roller, but make sure that the hair between the roller and scalp, which pulls directly on the root, is loose. Do this whether you use brush, plastic, or metal rollers. Foam-rubber rollers are less likely to cause hair loss because they don't pull the hair from the scalp as tightly. Brush rollers, however, are the most likely to cause hair breakage.

There is no evidence that metal clips or plastic clips cause hair loss or breakage under normal use. If bobby pins are used to hold rollers in place, they should be rubber tipped.

9

Excess Hair—Hirsutism

CAUSES OF EXCESS HAIR GROWTH

What causes excess hair growth, especially in girls and women?

Excess hair may be caused by many factors. It is most frequently an inherited characteristic common to either specific families or races of people. For instance, Mediterranean and Semitic people are more hairy than those of Nordic or Anglo-Saxon strains. In general, fair-skinned people are more hairy than blacks, while Orientals and American Indians are the least hairy.

Hair of abnormal texture, or increased amounts of hair in areas usually associated with little or no hair growth, is referred to as superfluous hair (hirsutism). There are many causes. Congenital hirsutism, which is present at birth or occurs early in childhood, is usually extensive; hair may even cover the body completely. Localized growth of hair in moles and birthmarks may occur at any time.

The above types of hirsutism are not related to the facial type that appears in females after puberty. Facial hirsutism involves a change in texture or an increase in the amount of hair on the chin, upper lip, and sides of the face. Most women with facial hirsutism have no related internal disturbance. The cause apparently is a matter of heredity or constitution, or part of normal growth and development. However, some cases of hirsutism are associated with glandular disorders, menopause, or side-effects from drugs as discussed in the following answers.

EXCESS HAIR AND HORMONES

I have read that excess hair may be caused by hormones and that treatment by a physician will correct the problem. Is this true?

Internal disorders, such as an imbalance in the secretion of hormones or the administration of certain medications, are infrequent causes of excess hair.

If you do not have a family tendency toward hairiness, and if an increase in undesirable hair has been relatively sudden or rapid, you should consult a physician. If an internal disorder is found and corrected, either by medical or surgical treatment, hair growth often returns to normal over a period of several months. If the hair growth pattern is well established some excess hair may persist, but it will not increase further.

EXCESS HAIR AS A SIDE-EFFECT

I have taken ACTH and related compounds for several years for rheumatoid arthritis. Suddenly I have developed a heavy growth of hair on my face. My doctor does not consider the condition serious, but I am becoming desperate. I have been bleaching this hair, but the growth is so heavy and long that bleaching is no longer effective. Is there anything else I can do?

Hirsutism is one of the side-effects of long-term administration of ACTH (corticotropin) and related compounds. In other cases, hirsutism may be inherited or may increase following menopause. Although hirsutism is not a serious threat to health, it can have serious psychological and cosmetic implications.

As long as drug administration continues, the problem

of excess hair cannot be permanently solved. However, various treatments can be helpful for making it less obvious. Electrolysis is the only satisfactory method for permanent removal of hair, but for your condition treatment would probably be long and expensive. One of the temporary measures discussed later in this chapter would be more practical.

SUPERFLUOUS FACIAL HAIR AT MENOPAUSE

I am disturbed by an increased growth of facial hair that began shortly after the start of menopause. Is such hair growth natural? Will this increased growth continue or is it temporary?

Hirsutism often appears after menopause but may sometimes appear before, mainly because of heredity. Hairs on the upper lip, the chin, and sides of the face become darker and thicker. While authorities differ as to exactly what causes this increased growth, it is not considered abnormal.

The trend toward increasing hairiness will continue, although for most women it reaches a plateau; it is not a relentless march to a full-blown beard. Various methods of removing or concealing the growth are discussed later in this chapter.

EXCESS FACIAL HAIR FROM USE OF CREAMS

Is it true that the use of cold cream will cause development of excess facial hair?

The belief that the use of cold cream and other emollient creams causes excess facial hair is evidently a common misconception among women.

A more logical explanation for this association is the fact that excess hair often appears before or during menopause, a time when dry skin often becomes more of a problem and creams are being used more frequently. Since creams are used on the same areas where excess hair begins to appear, the two may be incorrectly associated.

EXCESS HAIR IN CHILDREN

My dark-haired six-year-old daughter has a lot of body hair, especially on her arms and legs. My mother and sister also have dark, excessive body hair. Now other children at school are making unkind remarks about my daughter's hair. She is becoming very self-conscious. She insists on wearing tights all the time to cover her legs and long-sleeved dresses and blouses to cover her arms. What should I do? Can the hair be removed?

In the majority of cases, excess hair or degree of hairiness is an inherited characteristic. Children normally have a certain amount of body hair, although it usually does not increase and become evident until puberty. If this hair is dark-colored it will be more obvious than the same amount of light-colored hair. However, abnormal, excessive hair growth can occur in children. Such hair growth, if not an inherited trait, usually is related to an internal glandular disorder.

It appears that excessive hair is common in your family, but you should consult your pediatrician about your daughter's case if only for your own peace of mind. If the pediatrician believes that the amount of her hair is abnormal, consultation with another specialist such as a dermatologist or endocrinologist may be recommended. If this is an inherited characteristic, nothing can stop the hair growth. It may even increase somewhat after your daughter reaches puberty.

Cosmetic treatment of excess hair in young children is not recommended unless absolutely necessary. Such measures emphasize the problem, making the child even more aware of it. Instead, parents should play down the significance of the hair so that the child will accept it as normal and not be affected by the comments of other youngsters. In some cases, however, inattention to the condition may cause the child to become disturbed. Follow your physician's advice about treatment of your daughter's condition.

Of the various methods for removal or concealment of

excess hair, bleaching is most often recommended for children, but methods such as shaving or chemical depilatories may be used if indicated. If you decide to bleach your daughter's excess hair, a local beautician should be able to advise you about bleaching professionally.

Bleaching preparations for use at home are discussed later in this chapter.

METHODS OF REMOVING SUPERFLUOUS HAIR

What treatments are available for removing superfluous hair?

Superfluous hair may be concealed by bleaching, or removed by various methods such as tweezing (plucking), clipping, waxing, shaving, chemical depilation, and electrolysis.

The effects of all these methods except electrolysis are temporary and none is completely satisfactory. Each method has advantages and disadvantages. The choice of method depends on the character of the hair, the area and amount of growth, and personal preference.

Whether temporary methods tend to increase or distort hair growth is still controversial. Recent scientific studies indicate that these methods do not influence hair growth because they have no effect on the hair root, which determines the structure of the hair. These studies point out that temporary methods merely appear to thicken individual hairs because a short hair is less flexible than a long hair, and therefore feels more bristly (as illustrated by a short "crew cut" versus a long hair style).

With increasing age, superfluous hair tends to become darker and thicker, even if no attempts are made to remove it. Since hair removal methods usually are not employed until these changes begin to appear, the changes often are attributed to the methods.

However, trauma to the hair follicle from use of these

temporary methods sometimes results in a mild inflammatory reaction. When repeated often, it may eventually cause enough damage to shrink the follicles and thus appear to decrease hair growth or, instead, it may actually stimulate local hair growth.

HAIR REMOVAL BY X RAY

Are X-ray treatments safe and effective for removing excess hair?

Removing hair by X ray or any electrical ray of "special construction" is condemned at present. Many states specifically prohibit the use of X ray for this purpose by nonmedical persons. Other states require registration of all installations "in which radiation is intentionally administered to a human being for diagnostic or therapeutic purposes." However, some unsupervised nonmedical personnel and quacks still use radiation machines under a variety of names.

Cancer formation at the treatment sites may be a serious complication when radiation is used to remove hair. These cancerous changes may occur up to twenty years or more after the treatments are given.

BLEACHING SUPERFLUOUS HAIR

What are the pros and cons of bleaching for concealing excess hair?

Bleaching can make hair growth on the arms or upper lips less conspicuous. It may also be used in conjunction with temporary removal methods such as clipping. Bleaches are commercially available or may be prepared at home (see following answer).

Bleaching has certain advantages over other methods in that it is painless and usually does not harm the skin. Repeated bleaching also damages the hair, which then tends to break off. Its obvious disadvantage is that the hair is still present (although less obvious). Some people find that their skin is irritated by the bleaching process.

FORMULA FOR HOME BLEACH

What is the formula for making a bleach to conceal superfluous hair?

You can make your own preparation for bleaching using the following formula: Mix 6 percent hydrogen peroxide (known as 20-volume peroxide) with 20 drops of ammonia per 1 ounce of peroxide. Either household ammonia or ammonia water available at most drug stores can be used. If the freshly mixed bleach does not perform properly, the problem is probably (1) inactive, old peroxide or (2) insufficient ammonia.

Apply the bleaching preparation immediately after mixing because peroxide action begins as soon as the ammonia is added; leave it on for about half an hour. If your hair is not bleached enough with one application, the procedure can be repeated in a day or so.

Because skin irritation may develop in sensitive people, prepare a small amount of the bleaching solution and apply it to a small test area first. If irritation occurs within 30 minutes, the concentration of bleach as well as the length of time the application is left on should be reduced. A large volume of fresh bleaching solution required for the proposed bleaching application should be prepared after this initial test has been completed.

SHAVING EXCESS FACIAL HAIR

What do you think about shaving for removal of excess hair on the face?

Shaving is used more than any other method to remove underarm and leg hair, but most American women are repelled at the thought of shaving their faces; it seems too masculine. Perhaps surprisingly, there is no medical reason for not shaving to remove facial hair. Contrary to popular belief, shaving (like other methods of temporary removal) does not affect the texture, color, or rate of hair growth. The hair root, which determines the structure of hair, is located below the skin surface and is not affected by anything done to the dead hair shaft at or above the surface.

Temporary methods appear to thicken individual hairs because a short hair is less flexible than a long hair and therefore feels more bristly. Also, women who wish to remove superfluous hair usually do so at a time when more and thicker hair is appearing due to natural causes.

Shaving does have the disadvantage that it must be repeated every day or so to avoid a bristly feeling. Also, if the face is damaged by nicks and cuts from shaving the skin may look unattractive.

REMOVING SUPERFLUOUS HAIR WITH WAX

Is waxing a safe method for the removal of superfluous hair? What does it involve?

Waxing is one of the oldest methods of temporary hair removal and one of the least popular. It is most often used in this country to remove excess hair from facial areas such as the upper lip or chin. Many beauty parlors use waxing on the arms and legs, but this practice is more common in other countries.

In most cases the wax must first be heated. Then a layer of melted wax is applied to the skin, allowed to cool, and quickly stripped off in the direction of hair growth. Hairs are imbedded in the wax and plucked out as the wax is removed. A few "cold" waxes are available that do not require heating before use; the method of application and the results are the same as with warm waxes (a variation of waxing, called "zipping," is discussed later in this chapter).

Because hairs are plucked out below the surface, just above the root, the results of waxing are longer lasting. It generally takes several weeks for new growth to become evident. On the negative side, waxing may be painful and cause skin irritation, particularly when heated waxes are too hot when applied. Hairs must be long enough to become embedded in the wax, so for a short time the presence of some visible hair must be endured before the next waxing can be performed.

Although an increasing number of waxing preparations are available for home use, the technique of application and removal requires a certain amount of experience. Thus most waxing is done in beauty salons.

SAFETY OF CHEMICAL DEPILATORIES

Are chemical depilatories safe for removing superfluous hair from the legs and face?

Depilatories are used primarily for arm and leg hairs; they should not be used on the face unless specifically stated on the product's label. Also, they should never be used if there are breaks in the skin.

Although a few quick-acting (5 minutes or less) depilatories are now available, a depilatory generally takes 10 to 15 minutes to work on some areas of the underarms or legs. Many women consider this inconvenient; shaving is faster. Also, the products may have an unpleasant odor. On the other hand, using a depilatory does not have the masculine connotation of shaving.

It is claimed that the results of depilatories last longer than those of shaving because the hair is removed closer to the skin surface, but the difference (if it exists) is probably slight.

Chemical depilatories are available in foam, cream, or liquid form. Their effectiveness varies according to the type of hair growth. For instance, a thin hair is destroyed in shorter time than a thick hair. Depilatories may not be effective on some people and in some body areas without remaining on the skin for so long a time that skin irritation follows.

The first time you use a chemical depilatory, try it on a small area to familiarize yourself with the process. In some instances these products may cause skin reactions; if this happens, discontinue use of the product.

Follow package directions carefully; the manufacturer has included them to insure maximum safety and efficiency. Pay special attention to the length of time the preparation is to be left on your skin. The time is calculated so that the hair will be destroyed with minimum damage to your skin; this varies with different brands according to the chemical used and/or its concentration. Also follow the manufacturer's instructions concerning the time interval to be observed before a depilatory cream is reapplied to the same skin area.

AEROSOL DEPILATORIES

How effective are spray-on hair removers? Are they safe for underarms or just for legs?

Spray-on hair removers are simply chemical depilatories in aerosol spray form, and are promoted primarily for use on leg hair. Some manufacturers also suggest that their products be sprayed onto the hand first and then applied to the underarms. However, we do not advise their use in the underarm area. Check the label for special precautions and instructions regarding a specific product, and be careful not to accidentally spray any of the product into your eyes.

Commercial depilatories break down the structure of the hair so that it detaches easily from the skin at its surface. The composition of the hair and skin are similar, however, and any compound that has a destructive effect on hair will also affect skin—and may cause irritation.

Chemical depilatories supposedly remove hair closer to the skin surface than, for example, shaving does, thus providing longer lasting results, but the difference is hardly significant.

ABRASIVES FOR HAIR REMOVAL

I have seen advertisements for a device to remove super-fluous hair that looks like a small piece of stone. Do these things work?

The product is probably a pumice stone. Pumice, which is volcanic glass, can be ground into powder, then pressed into various solid shapes for use as an abrasive; other ingredients may be mixed with pumice powder to modify the texture. Pumice stones are used most often for removing rough skin on heels and elbows. Stones used for removal of excess hair generally have a smoother texture than those meant to be used on rough, thickened skin.

Abrasives such as pumice are among the oldest devices employed for temporary hair removal. Rubbing pumice over the skin generates mechanical friction, which wears off hairs at the skin surface.

These devices are inexpensive and easy to use, and are not as likely as chemical depilatories to cause skin irritation. They are, however, somewhat slow and tedious to use, and are impractical for large areas. If the abrasive is rubbed too vigorously, your skin will feel irritated. Once the hairs are removed, regular treatments thereafter may be less time consuming since the hairs will be short. Hair growth may become less coarse or dense after years of using a pumice; however, this procedure will not remove hair permanently.

After using a pumice it is advisable to gently massage a mild cream or lotion into the area to lessen any skin irritation produced by the abrasion.

OTHER METHODS OF TEMPORARY REMOVAL

What other methods are available for temporary removal of excess hair?

Plucking with tweezers is the preferred method for temporary removal of scattered hairs on the face or chest. It is obviously impractical when growth is extensive such as on legs and arms. Plucking may be somewhat painful, but has no other adverse effects. Regrowth sufficient to require repeated plucking may occur anywhere from 2 to 12 weeks, depending on the density and speed of hair growth in a given area. It is interesting to note that women do not hesitate to pluck eyebrow hairs but often believe it is harmful to pluck hairs elsewhere.

Clipping may be satisfactory for removing hairs from the upper lip and chest and has no disadvantages except that it is temporary.

PLUCKING AND HAIR GROWTH

Does plucking hairs make them grow back darker and coarser?

Scientific evidence does not substantiate this belief. For example, plucking eyebrows over the years seems to have little effect on their growth. If a hair has stopped growing and is waiting to be shed (hair grows in cycles) plucking it may stimulate a new hair to start growing right away—but in the same thickness and coarseness as before. On the other hand, some areas naturally change. An example is bushier eyebrows on men as they reach middle age compared with early adulthood.

PERMANENT HAIR REMOVAL—ELECTROLYSIS

What is electrolysis? Is it the only method of permanent hair removal?

The only safe way to permanently remove hair is by destroying the hair root with an electric current. A very fine wire needle is inserted into the opening of the hair follicle, and an electric current is transmitted down the needle. This destroys the hair root at the bottom of the follicle and loosens the hair, which then is removed from the follicle with tweezers.

This process uses either a galvanic current (electrolysis)

or a modified high-frequency electric current (electrocoagulation), but both types of current are commonly called electrolysis. The advantage of electrocoagulation is that more hairs can be removed in each session. Electrolysis is much slower, but the incidence of regrowth after treatment is lower. A newer system of electrolysis called photoepilation (destruction of the hair root by pulsed and guided light beam) appears to be limited in performance, at least with present equipment.

Because most professional machines today utilize the high-frequency current, some operators and salons advertise that they do not perform electrolysis, implying that they have a unique system of hair removal. Technically, they don't perform electrolysis. But the basic procedure and final results are essentially the same, regardless of the type of current or the brand of machine used. The safety and effectiveness of the technique depend primarily on the expertise of the operator, not on the machine.

Unfortunately, the competence of nonmedical electrolysis operators varies widely; many states have no standard training and licensing requirements. Few physicians do electrolysis themselves, but some have technicians trained in the technique or may refer patients to competent operators.

POTENTIAL DISADVANTAGES OF ELECTROLYSIS

Are any disadvantages and dangers associated with electrolysis treatments?

Electrolysis has a number of disadvantages and is not suitable for all cases of excess hair. It can be a long, tedious, expensive, and uncomfortable process. Cases of extensive hair growth may involve treatments (usually half an hour) once or twice a week for 1 or 2 years or longer, because each hair root must be treated individually. For this reason, electrolysis is generally recommended for removal of facial hair, while temporary methods are considered more practical for the arms and legs.

Excessive electric current, particularly high-frequency current, may damage skin around the hair follicle and result in scarring. Other, usually temporary complications are infections and spots of hyperpigmentation. Satisfactory results with minimal reactions and little danger of scarring are produced by using fine needles and the smallest amount of current that is effective, and by limiting the number of hairs removed in close proximity during each treatment. It is better to "thin out" the area than to concentrate on one spot. Also, it is normal to have some hairs present; if all are removed, wrinkling may occur later in life.

HAIR REGROWTH AFTER ELECTROLYSIS

Why do some hairs regrow after electrolysis if the procedure is supposed to be permanent?

A certain amount of hair regrowth always occurs after electrolysis, even when it has been performed by a skilled operator. Most experts estimate that 40 to 60 percent regrowth is normal; higher percentages are more common with electrocoagulation. Some hair growth recurs because the operator is working "blindly"; some follicles are crooked or grow at an angle, and it is not always possible to be certain that the needle has touched and destroyed the root. Also, the operator may use insufficient current to destroy the root in an effort to minimize discomfort and reactions. Since the hair is always plucked as part of the treatment, it is not possible to be sure immediately whether the hair has been temporarily or permanently removed. If the root has not been destroyed, the hair has simply been plucked and will regrow within several weeks and require treatment. If the root has been destroyed the hair should be removed very easily with tweezers, without exerting pressure or "plucking"; the unskilled operator may not be able to make this distinction.

Electrolysis destroys only the hair that is present; it has no effect on the cause of excessive hair growth. Also, at the time of treatment many hairs may be present but not visible because they have been manually removed by some temporary measure or have temporarily stopped growing (remember, hair grows in cycles). If hairs appear at approximately the same site as those that have previously been removed, the person may think they are treated hairs regrowing when they are actually other hairs.

PRACTICAL LIMITATIONS OF ELECTROLYSIS

Can electrolysis be used in all cases of excess hair?
Each case should be evaluated by a dermatologist to determine whether electrolysis is indicated. In some instances it may not be advisable. For example, since severe excess hair growth on the face may require weekly treatments for 3 to 4 years, the method would not be satisfactory for most teenage girls. For them a temporary method, repeated as often as necessary, would be better. For some, removal of facial hair might be so important that they would be willing to undergo prolonged treatment. However, the ideal patient for electrolysis is twenty to fifty years old and has grouped, bristly hairs on the chin or cheeks.

Any growths that contain hair, such as moles, must be diagnosed and evaluated by a physician before electrolysis is performed.

Removal of hair from thighs and arms by electrolysis is a long, tedious, and expensive procedure. Dermatologists usually discourage electrolysis for these areas; instead, they may suggest temporary methods such as shaving, waxing, or use of abrasives or chemical depilatories. Bleaching may satisfactorily conceal superfluous hair in these areas.

HOME METHODS OF HAIR REMOVAL

Can hair removal be done at home?
Most methods of temporary removal, as well as bleaching, can be carried out at home. However, the results of waxing are

usually better when the procedure is done by an experienced professional beauty operator. Home devices for electrolysis provide limited benefits, as the following answer points out.

HOME ELECTROLYSIS DEVICES

What is your opinion of the small, battery-operated electrolysis devices (epilators) that claim to remove excess hair safely and permanently?

Various types of home electrolysis devices are advertised for permanent hair removal. These devices, with slight variations, consist of a barrel or tube to be used as a handle and contain batteries to provide the electric source. A metal wire or needle extends from the barrel or from a cord and transmits the current. One device is designed with a retractable point so that the needle, when properly used, is less likely to penetrate the skin except at the opening of the hair follicle. Other devices require the user to locate the minute opening of the hair follicle to insert the needle. If the needle penetrates the skin instead of the hair follicle, the electric current may damage surrounding tissue. The basic procedure is the same as that used in professional electrolysis, and complications are also comparable. Except for cost, home electrolysis has all the disadvantages of the professional procedure, and more.

Inexperienced users may have more difficulty than a skilled professional operator in determining the direction of the hair follicle, the location of the root and the amount of current needed to destroy the root. More than one treatment will probably be required to destroy many hairs permanently. The time limit on the manufacturer's money-back guarantee may expire before the user determines she is satisfied with the device, since it may take several weeks—just as in professional electrolysis—to determine whether hairs have been permanently destroyed or simply plucked.

In contrast to professional treatments in which an experienced, skilled operator using a machine with a modified high-frequency current can remove several hundred hairs per session, the inexperienced operator of a home device will probably be able to remove no more than thirty to forty hairs per hour. Older people in particular may not be able to sustain use of the device for a long period.

A home device may be awkward and difficult to use for self-treatment of hair on the face, since it must be done before a mirror. In a mirror every movement is reversed, of course, so that an apparent move to the right is actually a move to the left. For this reason, home devices are better suited for removal of hairs from areas such as the lower arms and legs, which are readily accessible, while professional electrolysis is best for removing facial hairs.

The degree to which safe and satisfactory results are obtained from self-electrolysis treatments depends to a large extent on the condition of the user's hair and skin and the equipment used. If the user follows the manufacturer's directions carefully, with patience, time, and the development of skill, permanent removal of some hair by home electrolysis can be achieved.

HORMONE "ZIPPING" FOR HAIR REMOVAL

I have heard about an estrogen "zipping" method for permanent removal of excess hair. Is this treatment safe and effective?

The "zipping" procedure, which has been used for years to remove excess hair temporarily, is a variation of waxing. It consists of applying a thin layer of wax to the skin, followed by a cloth strip. After the wax has set, the strip is quickly "zipped" off the skin in the direction of hair growth. Hairs embedded in the wax are thus removed by the stripping action. The effects are the same as those of waxing, and ordinarily new growth does not become visible for several weeks.

This technique is generally a safe and effective means of

temporary hair removal. It can be somewhat painful, however, and skin irritation may develop, particularly if the wax is too hot when applied.

The rationale for adding topically applied female hormones (estrogens) to the zipping process is unknown. We are not aware of any scientific evidence to indicate that the use of estrogen creams in conjunction with zipping results in permanent hair removal. Furthermore, most cases of excess hair are not related to endocrinologic (hormonal) abnormalities. In the few cases that are, medical care is necessary.

SHAVING AND HAIR GROWTH

Does cutting or shaving have an effect on the rate of hair growth?

That cutting or shaving hair makes it grow faster is a popular belief, but one that has not been substantiated by scientific evidence. No apparent change in the numbers, thickness, or other characteristics of hair results from cutting or shaving.

Hair above the skin is essentially dead tissue and has no bearing on the growing part of the hair. Under certain abnormal conditions, however, local irritation can change the character or amount of hair growth. One example is the increased amount and thickness of hair under a plaster cast, where the skin is constantly pressed or rubbed for weeks or months at a time. This change is reversible in a short time after the cast is removed.

Occasionally, a woman will start to have thickening and darkening of facial hair, which then becomes more noticeable. This may occur normally in perfectly healthy women and is frequent during menopause. In rare cases it may be due to specific hormonal abnormalities.

Once increased growth and darkening have begun and are continuing, the woman may clip or shave these hairs and blame the continued increase and darkening on shaving, when actually shaving has played no role in changing the hair. Similar changes have been noted in women who have not shaved.

SHAVING THE LEGS

I would appreciate some advice on shaving my legs.
You can do several things to make leg shaving easier, safer, and cleaner.

When shaving with a razor blade, be sure your skin is wet. Wet hair is easier to cut because it is soft and pliable. Lathering with either soap and water or a shaving cream will facilitate the procedure.

Use a clean razor and a sharp blade. Blades used and discarded by men are usually too dull and cause discomfort and possible irritation.

Use long, even strokes rather than short, choppy ones. Rinse the blade frequently to remove cut hairs and soap foam. Shave your legs against the grain so that hairs are picked up before they are cut by the razor. When you shave with the grain, hairs tend to lie flat against the skin. Usually this means shaving with upward strokes, but studies have shown that the pattern of hair growth varies in different areas such as the back of the calves and the thighs.

Women who have diabetes, blood diseases, bleeding tendencies, skin rashes, or varicose veins should use extra caution to avoid irritation. Bony areas such as the ankle and shinbone are most susceptible to nicking, so use a razor lightly there. It is better to shave more frequently than too closely.

If you prefer an electric shaver, a preshave lotion helps remove unwanted perspiration that can interfere with the best shaving action of an electric razor.

Most nicks and scrapes caused by shaving are due to haste or carelessness. When bleeding occurs, apply pressure to the nick with a dry, clean cloth or tissue for a minute or two until the bleeding has stopped. A styptic pencil will serve the same purpose.

SHAVING THE THIGHS

My mother won't let me shave my upper legs, but I think they look terrible when I wear shorts or a swimsuit. What do you think? Is it harmful to shave this area?

Hairs on the upper legs that are dark-colored and obvious may present an undesirable appearance when shorts or bathing suits, especially bikinis, are worn.

Shaving hairs on the upper legs is not harmful. Chemical depilatories, wax depilatories or shaving may be used to remove the hairs temporarily. While it is popularly believed that cutting or shaving hairs makes them grow faster or become coarse and dark colored, scientific studies do not bear this out. No change in the numbers, thickness, or other characteristics of hair results from cutting, shaving, or other methods of temporary removal. Hairs appear more coarse and bristly as they grow out after shaving because short hair is less flexible.

Short, bristly hairs on the inner sides of the thighs may produce an uncomfortable feeling whenever the thighs rub together or when long-legged panty girdles or similar garments are worn. However, as the hairs grow longer, they become more flexible and the bristly feeling disappears. Some people may prefer temporary discomfort to the appearance of hairs.

Another approach that may conceal dark hairs satisfactorily is bleaching. Commercially prepared bleaching products are available from several cosmetic companies, or you can make your own preparation by adding a few drops of ammonia to 6 percent hydrogen peroxide. (See "Formula for Bleaching" earlier in this chapter for details.)

SUMMERTIME SHAVING

Every summer I have the same problem. When I wear a bathing suit, some pubic hair shows; if I shave, it itches. What can I do about this?

The itching is caused by two factors: the shaving procedure

itself and the regrowth of hair. To counteract the problem, always shave wet, not dry; use a sharp blade; take smooth, gentle strokes; and be generous with shaving cream or lather. Also, shave frequently—every day if necessary—to eliminate the sharp and bristly regrowth. (Too frequent shaving, however, can cause some skin irritation.)

After shaving, use emollient creams and lotions (but not alcoholic after-shave products) and dusting powders to help alleviate some of the discomfort.

REMOVING HAIR ON THE BREASTS

I have often noticed small hairs appearing around the outer edges of the nipples on my breasts. Are such hairs normal? Is it harmful to remove them? I would like to get rid of them permanently.

The presence of small hairs on this part of the breasts after puberty is normal. These hairs, along with other body hair such as underarm and pubic hair, are controlled by the sex hormones that become active at puberty. This growth of hair is similar to that which men develop on their chests. The amount of hair in either case depends primarily on heredity. Women who do not exhibit this hair most likely have removed it by one of the procedures discussed below.

If hair grows in excessive amounts or in areas where it usually is not present, consult a physician. Excess hair may be caused by certain internal disorders, such as hormonal imbalances, or by certain drugs. Diagnosis and treatment of the underlying cause (if one is found) will stop the increase in hair growth, and hair already present may slowly disappear. However, in most cases there is no abnormality and the excess hair is simply a genetic trait.

If you find the hairs undesirable, temporary removal by clipping, gentle shaving or plucking may be the most practical solution. None of these procedures is harmful, but plucking may be a little painful.

Electrolysis is the only permanent method of hair removal. When performed by a competent operator, electrolysis can be safely used for removal of breast hairs. It will not interfere with functioning of the mammary glands or produce cancer, tumors, or other ill effects.

TWEEZING HAIR FROM MOLES

I have a mole on my chin with a dark, coarse hair growing from it. Can I safely remove the hair from the mole by tweezing? Are there other safe methods of removal?

The hair in any mole becomes darker and coarser with time. Constant tweezing will not prevent future hair growth. Quite frequently, a small irritation will develop around hair follicles within the mole as a result of tweezing.

For temporary removal, the hair can be clipped close to the surface. Surgical removal of the mole will remove the pigmented lesion and the hair at the same time. A physician, or an electrologist under a physician's supervision, can also remove the hair permanently by epilation, leaving the mole untouched. Often, when this has been done the mole shrinks and becomes less noticeable. If you have any questions about the nature of the mole, it should be examined by a physician.

10

Shaving Advice for Men

WHICH SHAVE IS BEST?

Is any one method of shaving preferable to others?
Since little scientific research has been conducted on the effects of shaving, we are not sure whether one method is better than another.

No proof exists that any method is best for all skins. Individual preference among shaving methods is determined by such factors as hair and skin type, frequency of shaving, the presence of skin problems, and convenience.

However, one scientific study indicated that hair ends are ragged and split when shaved with an electric razor, while a blade razor leaves them smooth. The study also showed that with routine shaving the blade razor cuts hair closer to the surface and leaves a "stubble" of more uniform length. In practical terms, this means that a smoother, closer shave can be obtained with a blade razor.

FASTER SHAVING

What is the most effective beard softener in preparation for shaving? How can the length of time required to soften a beard be shortened?
The most effective beard softener in preparation for shaving is water. Beard hair softens in direct relation to its hydration

(water content). The time required for hydration and softening includes washing time, as well as the amount of time the shaving cream remains on the skin.

Washing your face with hot water prior to applying a shaving preparation is an easy way to shorten the time required to soften beard hair, since increased temperature causes quicker hydration. The shaving cream or soap may also help to increase hydration and will keep your beard softened. Usually 1½ to 2 minutes of contact with warm water is required for beard hair to become hydrated and softened.

INGROWN BEARD HAIRS

How does shaving cause ingrown hairs to develop? What can be done to prevent them?

Pseudofolliculitis (ingrown hairs) is one of the most frequent complaints in shaving. Several theories have been offered concerning its cause:

1. An inborn tendency to coarse, curly hair may cause closely cutoff ends of beard hairs to curve back and reenter the skin.

2. Shaving too close can result in clipping off whiskers beneath the skin surface. This may happen when men shave against the grain.

3. The smoothness or roughness of the cut edges of hairs may affect the production of ingrown hairs. The more roughened the edge, the more likely the hair is to catch in the skin and grow inward.

4. The duller the blade in wet shaving, the more pressure must be exerted and the greater the angle of the whisker's cut edge. A sharply angulated hair appears to have more chance of "curling" inward than growing outward.

If you are bothered by ingrown hairs, experiment to find the shaving method that gives you the least trouble. Don't shave against the grain; don't try to shave too closely (especially in the neck region); and use a sharp blade. Shave more often but not as closely.

If the problem of ingrown hairs is severe and persists in spite of all precautions, consult a physician to discuss the possibility of permanently removing the ingrowing hairs by electrolysis. Another alternative, of course, is to stop shaving altogether and grow a beard. Letting your beard grow during a vacation may be enough to solve the problem and allow irritation and secondary infection to clear up. Then shaving can be resumed.

INGROWN HAIRS—SPECIAL PROBLEM FOR BLACKS

Why is pseudofolliculitis such a problem for black men? Is there any alternative to shaving, since it aggravates the problem?

Pseudofolliculitis or "ingrown hair" is a serious problem for black men, and at times even for hirsute black women. The condition has its origin in the curved hair follicle of the black. Shaving produces a sharply pointed hair that reenters the skin. This causes a foreign-body reaction that results in abnormal scarring of skin. Shaving both causes and aggravates the condition. Growing a beard is one cure, though of course in some situations this may not be acceptable.

The best treatment involves avoiding any kind of razor (straight, safety and electric) and using chemical depilatories. In some cases electrolysis of at least the most affected regions of the beard is advisable.

Barium sulfide depilatories such as Magic Shave and others, therefore, have a definite place in the management of this affliction. In many people, however, the use of such depilatories produces an irritant contact dermatitis (rash). Physicians usually advise those with this problem to follow use of the depilatory with lukewarm wet dressings of water for a few minutes, then thorough soap-and-water washing, then application of a corticosteroid cream to allay the irritation. Most patients can work out an every-other-day shaving routine with one of the available depilatories.

WARTS AND SHAVING

What method of shaving is suggested for a man who has warts in the beard area?

A man with warts in the beard area should consult a physician promptly because the condition will persist or worsen. Many treatments are available for warts in this area: however, they can recur even after periods of seeming cure. There is no proof that any one method of shaving is better than another for a man with this problem. For more information on how warts are caused and can be treated, see Chapter 21, "Other Skin Problems."

PRESHAVE PREPARATIONS

Is it advisable to use a preshave preparation before shaving with an electric shaver? How about prior to wet shaving?

Preshave preparations are primarily used before shaving with electric shavers, but preshave preparations for wet shaving are also available. Their main purpose is to facilitate shaving and to reduce skin irritation associated with shaving procedures.

Preshave preparations for use before wet shaving are intended to "wet" and soften the beard to some degree before the application of shaving cream. The products may contain soap or a synthetic detergent and other agents to accelerate the wetting action in hard water. Somewhat similar results may be obtained by use of a shaving cream followed by a waiting period of a few minutes, then reapplication of the shaving cream before shaving.

In contrast to wet shaving, where the beard is first softened with water, the beard must be as dry as possible prior to electric shaving. Electric shaving should be preceded by removal of perspiration and oily secretions to prevent the beard from being slippery and elusive to the cutting edge of the electric razor. Effective preshave preparations help stiffen and raise individual hairs so that they can be caught between the razor's combs and removed.

Preshave preparations for electric shaving require the following: adequate astringency to stiffen the beard, quick drying to insure rapid evaporation of any moisture on the face, a slightly acid pH to prevent swelling of hairs, ability to provide a skin coating on which the razor will glide to minimize skin irritation, and the absence of ingredients that will corrode the cutting head or adversely affect the plastic parts of the electric shaver.

Preshave preparations are either astringent or oily. Astringent lotions have a higher concentration of alcohol and aim primarily at drying and stiffening the hairs. The astringent effect may be increased by adding other mild astringent agents. Lotions of the oily type aim primarily at lubricating the beard by depositing a thin oily film on the face. It is claimed that this will prevent the drag of the cutting head against the skin (especially troublesome in warm and humid weather).

SHAVING PREPARATIONS

How do various types of shaving preparations differ in composition and performance?
The major types of shaving preparations include soaps, lather creams, brushless shaving creams, and aerosol foams. All of these except brushless creams are basically soap preparations and produce lather.

A good shaving preparation should soften hairs quickly and hold them erect so that they can easily be cut. The product must remain stable when stored under normal conditions. Lather products should quickly produce a copious lather that does not dry out or collapse during the normal shaving time. It should not cause skin or mucous membrane irritation.

Soaps were the first shaving preparations but are used less today. The lather produced is plentiful, dense, and long lasting. Their disadvantage is that they have to be applied with a brush to produce lather in sufficient quantity.

Lather shaving creams are similar to soaps in formulation, with the addition of a humectant (moisture retaining agent) for softer consistency and for maintaining moisture in the lather. Different types of oils are added for foam stability and lubrication. Lather shaving creams are more convenient to use than soaps and are preferred by many men, but they also must be applied with a brush to produce sufficient lather.

Brushless shaving creams are similar in appearance to lather type creams, but are formulated quite differently. They are modifications of vanishing cream (an oil-in-water mixture) to which wetting agents, humectants, and other ingredients may be added. Brushless creams contain little or no soap, so they do not lather. The expressed cream is simply applied to the face, which is then shaved in the usual manner. A slight oily film remains after shaving, which is claimed to make the skin feel softer and less irritated. However, moistening and softening of the hairs takes longer than with a lather cream. So it may be necessary either to use a preshave preparation or to wash the face with soap and water before applying a brushless cream, in order to soften the beard sufficiently to obtain a comfortable shave.

Brushless shaving creams are traveling aids, since they don't require a brush and mug and there is no danger of the preparation discharging into shaving kits or luggage as may happen with aerosol foam preparations.

Aerosol foam shaving creams are the most recent development in shaving preparations. These products are basically a mixture of lather cream in liquid form with the addition of propellants, vegetable waxes and various oils. Their chief advantage is ease of application, and their effects are similar to those achieved with other lather shave preparations.

For men with "normal" skin, the choice of shaving preparations is a matter of personal preference. Shaving creams preferred for dry and oily skin are discussed in the following answer.

WHICH SHAVING CREAM IS BEST?

What kind of shaving cream should be used on oily skin? On dry skin?

Men with dry or soap-sensitive skin should use a brushless cream, which provides the most lubrication. Brushless creams are emulsions of oil in water, and will not rob the skin of its oils. However, washing the face thoroughly after shaving can contribute to dryness, as can the use of after-shave lotion. An emollient used after washing the face instead of after-shave lotion will counteract this dryness.

Men with oily skin would do best to choose either a lather-type shaving cream used with a brush or an aerosol foam. These creams are actually soaps, and tend to flush away oil better than brushless creams, which have a far lower soap content. A mentholated cream will also help because menthol has a degreasing action on the skin. Thorough washing after shaving, as long as it is not excessive, is beneficial for oily skin.

HOT SHAVING CREAMS

Is there any advantage in using "hot" aerosol shaving preparations that provide a warm shaving lather?

The theory behind hot shaving creams appears to be that heat helps to soften hairs, making shaving easier. Dry whiskers are hard, and a good deal of pressure is required to cut them, so the objective of a wet shave is to soften the whiskers. Hair will absorb water, and as it does it becomes soft and easier to cut. Heat improves the softening action and shortens the time required for the beard to soften. According to shaving authorities, thorough soaking of the hair is one prerequisite for ease in shaving.

Of course, thoroughly washing and rinsing the face in hot water or applying a hot, wet towel for a few minutes will achieve the same result as "hot" aerosol shaving preparations. On the other hand, "hot" aerosol lather is convenient and psychologically pleasant. A self-heating, "hot" shaving lather may have a definite advantage when hot water is not available on hunting, camping or fishing trips.

AFTER-SHAVE PREPARATIONS

What are the differences among men's colognes, after-shave lotions, and skin bracers or refreshers?
There is little difference between after-shave lotion and bracer or refresher products since their formulas are similar. They consist primarily of alcohol, water, and scent, with formulas differing according to the use intended.

An after-shave preparation is usually applied only to the face. It feels refreshing and may soothe razor discomfort. However, it is doubtful that any of these preparations has a therapeutic effect on the skin. The use of after-shave lotion is purely a cosmetic preference.

A skin bracer or refresher has a higher alcohol content than after-shave lotion and is used as a body refresher after a bath or shower. It may also be used as an after-shave lotion.

Cologne is a blend of selected essences and is lighter in scent than an after-shave lotion or bracer. It is used primarily for the scent rather than for any local effect on the skin.

11

Hair Loss—Baldness

NORMAL HAIR LOSS

I'm worried that I may become bald. Every day I find hairs on my pillow, in the wash basin, and on my brush and comb. What can I do to stop this hair loss?

A healthy scalp normally loses a certain number of hairs each day. It is also natural for a healthy scalp to start growing a number of hairs each day. Each human scalp hair has its own life cycle: a long growth period (normally from 2 to 6 years) followed by a much shorter resting period (usually about 3 months) in which the hair stops growing, separates from the root, and becomes club-shaped at the scalp end.

Club hairs slowly move upward and are easily dislodged by washing, brushing, and combing. Some people mistakenly think that the club-shaped end of the hair is the root and that this hair is lost permanently.

After a variable rest period, a new hair normally forms in the hair follicle, initiating a new growth cycle. If the old hair is still present, the new hair will push it out. The average daily rate of hair growth is 1/72 inch; therefore it takes about 2½ months for scalp hair to grow 1 inch.

Usually about 15 percent of the hairs scattered throughout the scalp are in the resting stage and gradually shedding; these are the hairs that you find on your pillow, in the wash basin, and on your brush and comb.

The normal daily rate of loss is twenty to sixty hairs. Only when the rate of loss exceeds the rate of new growth do thinness and balding become apparent. As a person grows older, the rate of loss exceeds the rate of new growth. Thus, some permanent thinning of hair is inevitable with age. Authorities estimate that 40 percent of a person's hair must be lost before thinness becomes evident.

If you feel your hair is thinning excessively, consult a dermatologist. In a few cases, other factors may cause excessive hair loss, as discussed in the following questions and answers.

BRUSH ROLLERS AND BALDNESS

Can brush rollers or ponytail and pigtail styles contribute to baldness?

Both tight plaiting of hair and the use of brush rollers have been blamed for causing bald spots on the scalp. When hair is regularly plaited, localized areas of hair loss sometimes develop where the hair is pulled most tightly. There have also been reports of bald spots with styles, such as ponytails and pigtails, that place hair under severe tension. This hair loss is seen more commonly along the front of the scalp, where the hair is under the greatest tension; some hairs have been pulled out, others broken off. Such loss occurs only after long-term use of these styling methods; it is not caused by their occasional use.

Brush rollers are popular because they produce an extremely tight curl, but they have been blamed for some cases of partial hair loss. The mechanism involved is probably similar to that discussed above; loss of hair follows prolonged, very tight curling. It is doubtful that occasional use will cause any significant hair loss.

Bald spots that result from plaiting, styling and the use of brush rollers are usually temporary. Hair normally regrows several months after the practice of placing the hair under excessive tension is stopped. This hair loss is known as traction alopecia and results from temporary injury to the growing end of the hair.

TRACTION ALOPECIA

I have developed some hair loss from wearing my hair tightly pulled back. Will this hair loss be permanent?

Pulling on hair, either from habit or to achieve certain hair styles, will cause a loss referred to as traction alopecia. Most of the hair will probably regrow because the roots are not destroyed. However, it has been observed that repeated or prolonged traction may cause some degree of permanent loss.

PREGNANCY AND HAIR LOSS

What causes hair loss after pregnancy and what can be done to prevent further loss?

This type of hair loss is common, and is related to the many changes that occur in the body during pregnancy and for a time after delivery. It is temporary, and hair growth returns to normal in a few months.

There is no specific therapy. Until the condition corrects itself, manipulate your hair as little as possible; brush with a soft, natural-bristle brush; shampoo gently with a mild shampoo; pat your hair dry instead of rubbing it; and avoid hair styles that either in setting or combing out pull your hair excessively.

HAIR LOSS AND "THE PILL"

Can oral contraceptives cause hair loss?

Mild hair loss of the scalp has been observed in some women taking oral contraceptives. It is usually temporary and regrowth generally takes place within several months after use of "The Pill" is discontinued. This loss is comparable to hair loss in true pregnancy discussed in the previous answer.

UNUSUAL BALDNESS

Our son, age twelve, has been losing his hair and is now bald. What could be the cause and what can be done?

The most probable cause of total hair loss in an otherwise healthy child is an extensive form of a disorder known as alopecia areata.

This type of hair loss often begins as rapidly appearing round bald spots on the scalp. These spots can enlarge as surrounding hairs loosen and shed. In most cases only one or a few spots appear, and hairs stop falling out after a few weeks. However, the disease may progress and the hairless areas merge to result in total baldness. In some cases hair may also be lost on other parts of the body.

In most patients with the limited, patchy form of alopecia areata, hair regrows spontaneously after several months. New hairs may at first lack pigment and have a finer texture than usual, but eventually they become entirely normal. Even in extensive forms of the disease, full, spontaneous regrowth may occur even after several years of baldness.

Alopecia areata is more likely to persist: (1) the more extensive it is, (2) the earlier in life it begins, and (3) the longer it is present. In cases of extensive or persistent hair loss, the most practical cosmetic management is the use of a wig or hairpiece.

The fundamental cause of alopecia areata is unknown. It is believed that the tissue is unable to tolerate pigmented hairs. The disorder is not contagious; it does have a moderate tendency to recur. In some cases, emotional stresses seem to precipitate or aggravate the condition. It has no cure, but in the majority of patients hair regrowth occurs. In some cases physicians can induce regrowth with the use of steroids; the method of administration is determined by size, extent, and duration of the lesions.

HAIR LOSS CAUSED BY ILLNESS

I recently recovered from a severe illness and my hair has become much thinner. Every time I brush it, more falls out. One doctor said my hair was thinning, but another said it was breaking off close to the scalp. What do you think? Will this condition be permanent?

Temporary hair loss is fairly common following severe illness accompanied by a high fever. Other factors that may contribute to temporary loss of hair include severe weight loss, certain medications, general anesthesia, X-ray therapy of the head and childbirth.

Any situation that adversely influences the body's metabolism or endocrine status will contribute to hair loss by increasing the number of hairs in the resting phase of the growth cycle. Human hairs grow in cycles, with a long period of growth followed by a short resting phase in which the hair stops growing and is shed. In a few months a new cycle begins and the lost hair is replaced.

Some illnesses may also cause hair to become dry and brittle and to break off close to the scalp. The same thing may occur from excessive bleaching and improper permanent waving. This situation is usually temporary and does not affect hair growth; the damage is limited to the dead hair shaft above the surface of the skin. New, undamaged hair will grow out to replace the damaged hair that has broken off. Since hair grows only about 1/72 inch per day, or 1 inch every 2½ months, the new growth may not become evident for several months.

Close examination of your hair by a dermatologist will indicate whether it is simply broken off or there is temporary loss, or both.

There is no specific therapy for hair loss following illness. Excessive vigorous manipulation of your hair should be avoided; this only leads to further hair damage and loss. Also, your hair should not be stretched, pulled on tight rollers, or worn in styles that pull it. Balanced nutrition, with an adequate protein intake, is essential for good hair growth, but we know of no specific vitamin(s) that will increase the rate of hair growth or strengthen hair.

BALDNESS IN MEN

What causes male pattern baldness and why is it so common? What progress has been made in preventing or curing this type of baldness?

Male pattern baldness (MPB) is found in sufficient degree to be of cosmetic significance in about 12 percent of men aged 25, 37 percent of men aged 35, 45 percent of men aged 45, and about 65 percent of men aged 65, increasing only slightly thereafter.

Androgen, a common term for male sex hormone, causes male pattern baldness in genetically predisposed individuals. The genes for MPB are inherited equally from the father's and mother's sides of the family. The extent of baldness and age of onset vary from family to family and from one individual to another within a family.

Since a man may inherit genes for MPB from both sides of his family, he may be more bald at a given age than either his father or his maternal or paternal grandfather or uncles. On the other hand, he may inherit baldness genes from only one side of his family, the other side lacking this hereditary trait, and thus he may be less bald than any of his male forebears at a comparable age.

Exactly how androgen causes male pattern baldness is not understood, but research is continuing and the cellular mechanisms will some day be defined.

Hairs grow in cycles. Each scalp hair grows for two to six years and then rests for about three months. After the rest period, the old hair comes out and a new hair grows from the same root. These cycles are repeated throughout life with individual hairs on different cycles. At any given time, approximately 85 percent of the hairs on a scalp are in the growing phase and 15 percent in the resting phase.

The hair cycle is important in male pattern baldness because the effect of androgen seems to be to shorten the growing phase—that is, the hair no longer grows for 2 to 6 years but for a shorter time, and each successive cycle becomes shorter. The man with MPB notices his hair becoming thinner and shorter. Later he notices that the hair on top of his head is failing to grow to any appreciable length. Finally, only a short growth of fuzz is seen. These short, difficult to see hairs are growing from roots that originally produced the long, thick hairs of former days. The roots keep repeating cycles of growth and rest, and may do so for ten, twenty, or more years. Only toward the end of this period are some of the roots actually lost.

Even the baldest scalp (due to MPB) contains tiny follicles that produce tiny, almost visible hairs. Further biological research may make it possible to keep the roots in the growing phase for a longer time, thereby slowing down the progression of baldness. However, it is extremely unlikely that a significant amount of hair will ever be grown on a bald scalp when that baldness has been caused by MPB. The victim of MPB can seek refuge in one of several hair replacement techniques discussed later in this chapter.

BALDNESS IN WOMEN

I am a woman of fifty-five, and for the last year or so I have been losing a lot of hair. What can I do to stop this hair loss?

Women often develop thinning of the hair with age. In some this may become quite pronounced at middle age or later. It is not associated with any disease, but seems to be the same type of condition as male baldness, although it does not progress to the same extent. The pattern of hair loss may resemble that of male baldness, with a receding hairline and some thinning at the top of the scalp. Little can be done to alter this type of hair loss; but most women retain enough hair to provide adequate cosmetic coverage.

Within recent years, complaints from women of more generalized hair loss at an earlier age appear to have increased markedly. The cause of this loss is not known. Factors such as sharp bristles in some nylon hair brushes, rollers that pull the hair tight, and certain hair styles such as tight twists that exert tension on the hair have caused hair loss in some cases. If hair is bleached excessively, it can become harsh and strawlike. Extensive hair breakage is not uncommon. If the cause is removed, the hair will usually regrow in a few months.

Temporary hair loss and thinning may occur occasionally following a surgical procedure, childbirth, or diseases in which there has been a high fever. Regrowth occurs within a few months in most cases.

There is no specific therapy for diffuse or temporary hair loss. To minimize further loss due to mechanical factors, avoid excessive manipulation of your hair, brush it moderately with a soft brush, shampoo regularly and gently with a mild shampoo, dry wet hair by letting the towel soak up the moisture rather than by vigorous toweling, and avoid hair styles that in setting or in combing out require excessive pulling of your hair.

Some cases of diffuse hair loss are associated with endocrine disorders such as hypothyroidism, other internal disorders or the administration of certain drugs. In such cases, treatment is directed at the underlying condition.

DIET AND HAIR LOSS

Is hair loss, luster, or texture affected by vitamin or diet deficiencies?

Nutritional deficiencies have not been shown to cause ordinary baldness. However, severe deficiencies of certain vitamins due to dieting or to severe digestive system disturbances may contribute to dryness, lack of luster, and, under conditions of chronic starvation, some hair loss. Constant dieting (especially if protein intake is inadequate) will influence size, composition, and growth of hair.

No single vitamin has been shown to have any pronounced influence on hair growth. If you believe you have a vitamin or other nutritional deficiency, consult your physician. Self-administration of vitamins, particularly excessive intake of Vitamin A, can have toxic effects.

HAIR WASHING AND BALDNESS

Can washing hair too often cause premature hair loss? My husband washes his hair every day, and it has become dry and brittle. Also, his hairline is receding and premature baldness seems to be setting in.

Excessive washing may cause hair to dry out because natural oils are removed. Dry, brittle hair may break off close to the scalp, simulating baldness. There is no evidence, however, that washing alone can cause baldness; on the other hand, daily washing does nothing to prevent baldness. Your husband probably is experiencing the normal male pattern baldness characteristic of many men. There is no known way to prevent this normal type of baldness.

DANDRUFF, OILY HAIR, AND BALDNESS

Can dandruff and oily hair cause baldness in men?

Any serious scalp disease is a threat to good hair health. However, scientific research has uncovered no evidence that dandruff and oily hair cause male pattern baldness. These are related only in one respect: the endocrine status that controls the production of oil also influences dandruff and hair loss.

At least 95 percent of all cases of male baldness are classified as normal male pattern baldness, for which there is no cure. Claims that preparations or treatments will cure male

pattern baldness by eliminating oily hair or dandruff should
be viewed with skepticism.

FRAUDULENT BALDNESS CURES

*Advertisements indicate that certain treatments will re-
grow hair on bald heads. Of what value are these treatments?*

Don't waste your money! Hair treatments and remedies claim-
ing to prevent, postpone, or correct baldness have been promoted for centuries, and they all have one thing in common—
they fail to grow hair.

The most common type of baldness, "male pattern baldness," probably accounts for 95 percent of all cases. It has a
characteristic pattern and course, progressing slowly over several years. The hair follicle gradually shrinks and finally produces a colorless hair only a few millimeters long. Since no
known drugs, remedies or external devices will replace hair
follicles, this type of baldness is considered permanent and
incurable. Although the exact cause is not known, sex, age,
and heredity are involved, and there isn't anything we can do
about any of them.

There are other kinds of baldness, but most of these are
temporary. Only personal, on-the-spot examination and diagnosis by a competent physician can determine the cause and
possible treatment of hair loss in these cases. The so-called
"hair and scalp specialists" often use before-and-after pictures
of persons who have suffered from a temporary form of baldness as a gimmick to attract customers. The deception lies in
the fact that in such cases regrowth would have occurred without treatment.

In spite of numerous actions by government agencies and
campaigns by health and consumer organizations, advertising
for worthless preparations and devices continues, and the public spends huge sums of money on them each year. Don't join
this group of victims.

NO ANTIBALDNESS SHAMPOO

Some shampoos promise to replace hair proteins or amino acids, thereby retarding hair loss. Is there any scientific evidence to support such claims?

Many ointments, shampoos, and other concoctions promise to perform miracles in preventing the loss of scalp hair, or even to "restore" a good growth of hair on bald scalps.

These claims are false. Such products can be placed in the same category as the treatments discussed in the previous answer. They have no effect on baldness.

TESTOSTERONE OINTMENT FOR BALDNESS

I have heard that baldness can be cured by applying an ointment containing testosterone to the head. What information do you have about this treatment?

Much publicity was given a few years ago to an experimental treatment involving the topical application of preparations containing the male hormone, testosterone, to balding heads. Evidently this caused many people to think that a cure for baldness had finally been found, and that commercial preparations for this purpose were available.

The use of testosterone to treat baldness is based on an experimental study by two physician-investigators. By anointing hairless areas of the scalp with testosterone cream, the investigators successfully rekindled a scraggly bit of hair growth in a few of the experimental subjects.

In a published report on the treatment in the *Journal of the American Medical Association*, the authors were quick to point out that this did not mean testosterone ointments are a cure for baldness. The regrowth of hair was minimal and scanty. Furthermore, testosterone may be readily absorbed through the skin and can produce unwanted side-effects. At present, these side effects have not been evaluated; therefore the ointments can be used only experimentally.

The authors stated in their report:

We know only too well that bald people grasp at hairs and cherish every fiber. They are ready to be gulled, deceived and deluded. We are fearful of the misinterpretation and mis-application of this work in the face of such intense feeling. We would strongly counsel against the indiscriminate use of testosterone. This is a potent hormone and its long-term use in an unsupervised population is to be condemned. Its use in females of reproductive age is obviously ruled out.

They added: "We do not regard that we have achieved a useful treatment for common baldness by topical administration of testosterone." Attempts by other investigators to duplicate the results obtained by the original researchers have been unsuccessful. At this time, no safe, effective topical treatment for baldness has been found.

HAIR TRANSPLANTATION

I would appreciate some information on the current status of hair transplantation.

Hair transplantation is a surgical treatment for male pattern baldness (MPB) that is usually performed in a physician's office with the patient awake, sitting up or lying down. In this procedure, a section of hair from the side or back of the scalp (areas not subject to MPB) is lifted up and the hair directly below is clipped short with scissors. The donor site (the clipped area) is cleansed and a local anesthetic is injected. The recipient site (the front or top of the scalp) is also cleansed and anesthetized.

Cylinders of skin 3 to 5 millimeters in diameter (4mm = 5/32 inch) are taken from the donor site. Each cylinder (graft) contains twelve to eighteen hair roots. Cylinders from the recipient site are removed and discarded. The donor grafts are then placed in the recipient holes following the normal angle of hair growth for that area. Although stitches, tapes, and glues have been used to hold the grafts in place, most physicians now allow nature to "glue" them in.

Following grafting, a nonstick dressing is usually applied to the donor and recipient areas. This is held in place overnight by a gauze wrap around the back of the head and forehead. It usually is removed the next morning, and the patient carefully combs his hair over the donor area to obscure the sites. A bandage on the transplants may or may not be needed. For the man wearing a hairpiece, a special tape or dressing may be placed over the grafts so that the hairpiece can still be worn.

Immediately following transplantation, care must be taken not to mechanically disturb the transplants. Their secure attachment to the scalp takes about two weeks, and vigorous activity should be avoided during that time.

The transplanted grafts form dark scabs that fall out in two to three weeks. After an additional one to two weeks, most if not all of the remaining transplanted hairs fall out, leaving bare, smooth spots. Two to 6 months later new hairs begin to grow, retaining the characteristics of hairs in the donor site. They grow at approximately the normal rate—slightly less than one-half inch per month.

Donor sites heal within two weeks after transplantation. Because these sites shrink during the healing process, overlying and surrounding hair covers them, so a large number of transplants can be obtained without creating obvious bare spots. However, new hairs do not grow in these spots; the total number of hairs on the head remains the same or slightly less.

Since not all of the grafts required can be put in at once, several grafting sessions are necessary. Transplants can be performed on a weekly or even shorter schedule, providing the grafts are put into different areas. Generally ten to twenty grafts are performed at one session, and sessions usually require 60 to 90 minutes each. Scheduling of sessions is adjusted to the patient's and physician's desires.

The total number of transplants needed depends on the amount of baldness, the abundance of donor hair, and the patient's capacity to tolerate the procedure (pain is usually mild and scarring is minimal). The average number of grafts required is 150 to 200; a minimum of 100 usually is needed to show any improvement, while patients fully bald may require 200 to 400 or more.

Transplanted hair may be dyed, combed, curled, or manipulated in any reasonable manner, but "crew cuts" are not suitable because scars can be seen more readily when not covered by surrounding hair.

Hair transplantation is not suitable for all cases of baldness, and the degree of success varies from one patient to another. The advantages of this hair replacement method over others are: (1) it is the only procedure that utilizes a person's own hair and provides results that last for virtually a lifetime; and (2) while the initial costs are high, they are one-time costs.

If you consider hair transplantation, select your physician carefully and ask to be shown photographs of patients treated previously. Do not have this procedure performed by a lay person.

Ideally, hair transplantation should be initiated at a time when hair loss has not progressed too far. Transplants can then be added in small numbers, as needed, with minimal cosmetic problems.

HAIR WEAVING

What is hair weaving? Is it safe and effective? Where can I go for treatment?

This procedure, merchandised mainly for men, provides a semipermanent hairpiece. The client must have some natural hair growth, which is used to form woven or braided base sections (anchor areas). Hairs or tufts of hair from stock supplies are sewn, woven, knotted, or cemented to the anchor areas. The hair is then trimmed and styled to blend with the client's own hair.

The results of this procedure in skilled hands can be excellent. The negative features are: (1) as the anchor hair grows, the entire hairpiece moves away from the scalp and needs to be retightened every 4 to 8 weeks; (2) this incurs repeated costs for as long as the weave is maintained; (3) cleansing the scalp is more difficult; and (4) in some cases, the tension created by tight braiding of the anchor hair produces traction alopecia (temporary baldness), such as results from wearing tight pigtails or from breakage.

If you decide that hair weaving is suitable for you, first try to determine the success of the agency you are considering. Ask to see satisfied customers or their pictures. Second, find out how long the agency has been in the community and plans to be there. The initial work should be performed at an agency expected to be in business for a long time, since the weave will require retightening every 4 to 8 weeks. Finally, check the number of complaints (if any) filed against the agency with local Better Business Bureaus. Hair weaving is a complex procedure requiring special skills, and should therefore not be undertaken lightly.

HAIR IMPLANTATION

How does hair implantation compare with other hair replacement techniques?

This hair replacement technique, known by many names, consists basically of sewing a hairpiece to the scalp. Stitches or other types of anchor points are inserted in the scalp by a physician. Later a technician, usually at a cosmetic shop, attaches a hairpiece or tufts of hair to the stitches.

Although this procedure seems to provide "instant hair," many problems exist. Often the body tolerates poorly stitches or wires left in place for prolonged periods of time. Unlike pierced ears, the scalp reacts violently. Redness, soreness, pus,

and infection may result. Continuous discomfort is not uncommon, and in some cases is so severe that resting the head
on a pillow becomes intolerable. When infection or a pus
reaction sets in, the sutures work out quickly and may leave
disfiguring scars.

If no scalp reaction occurs, daily combing and styling of
the hairpiece will result in the stitches eventually pulling out.
Research has shown that this often happens after 1 year, but
occasionally it takes as long as 3 years. Another disadvantage
of implantation is that cleaning beneath the sewed-on hairpiece is very difficult, and often an unpleasant odor develops.

Although many physicians have tried to perfect the procedure, hair implantation is still beset by numerous problems
and available evidence indicates that solutions are not immi-
nent. Before deciding on what many skin specialists consider
the least desirable approach to baldness, weigh the hazards
discussed above against the potential benefits.

HAIRPIECES

*I am considering buying a hairpiece. What information
can you give me about them?*

There are different types of hairpieces, and variations exist in
their quality and in the skill of the persons preparing them.
Among factory-made hairpieces, the difference between a good-
looking product and one that is obviously a hairpiece depends
on the skill of the person cutting, trimming, thinning, tinting,
and fitting your selection.

In general, you should become familiar with the basic
types of hairpieces:

1. The hard top is a hard plastic base into which hairs are
inserted. The types and shapes of plastic vary, as well as the
number of holes to improve ventilation. This type of hairpiece
usually maintains its shape better and has a longer life. Negative features are that it is heavier and may be uncomfortable in
warm, humid climates.

2. The soft mat consists basically of a synthetic fiber mesh as a base to which hairs are tied. The soft mat frequently is more comfortable in hot, humid climates, but usually loses shape faster and does not last as long as the hard top.

3. The front lace features a specially treated transparent synthetic mesh that extends slightly forward from the main body of the hairpiece. When properly glued to the front of the scalp, it is difficult to see under normal circumstances. This type of hairpiece requires extra time for careful application, and generally requires more care than the other types.

4. The partial piece is available in many varieties. A small net is used to give good coverage of limited areas.

You also need to decide on the type of hair to be used in your hairpiece. Natural hair is more expensive and requires coloring as often as every 6 or 8 weeks depending on sun exposure, but generally looks more natural. Synthetic hair is less expensive initially and involves less cost in terms of upkeep.

Don't buy the first hairpiece you see. Shop and compare. Examine the different types of hairpieces and the differences between natural hair and synthetic fibers. Determine whether hair styles suitable for your face can be easily accomplished with the hairpiece you prefer. Check the reputation of the seller through friends, former customers, or local Better Business Bureaus. Examine warranties and find out what recourse is available if you are not satisfied with the hairpiece. Finally, select a hairpiece that not only meets your physical needs but your personality and lifestyle.

WIGS AND HAIR LOSS

Does the frequent wearing of wigs and hairpieces cause hair to fall out and stop growing?

Frequent wearing of wigs and hairpieces has not been shown to cause hair to fall out or stop growing. Wearing a wig may occasionally cause increased perspiration, dandruff, and itching, which may be remedied by shampooing.

12

Other Hair Problems

DANDRUFF—SIMPLE AND SEVERE

What causes dandruff? Is seborrheic dermatitis a type of dandruff?

Dandruff is usually defined as a condition of itching and flaking of the scalp that appears 2 to 4 days after each shampoo. Everyone experiences this to some degree, and the point at which it becomes a source of annoyance is a matter of personal sensitivity. The minimal scaling of dandruff can usually be controlled by washing at proper intervals or by using one of the commercial preparations available for this purpose.

Occasionally dandruff symptoms become quite severe, and there may be redness and inflammation together with itching and flaking of the scalp. These symptoms may also appear in other areas—the sides of the nose, around the ears, or on the chest. Dermatologists refer to this condition as seborrheic dermatitis, and it usually calls for the attention of a physician.

If dandrufflike symptoms persist, always consult your doctor. Some diseases similar to dandruff do not respond to home treatments intended for dandruff (psoriasis is one).

Why scalp flaking becomes a problem for some but not for others is not known. Enough people want to prevent it, however, for manufacturers to have filled the marketplace with a great variety of lotions, tonics, and creams designed to meet the demand for a cure or alleviation.

Although microorganisms may contribute to the more

severe cases with secondary infection, it has never been shown that they cause dandruff. Some manufacturers have nevertheless tried to develop a treatment based on the hypothesis that dandruff is infectious in nature. These products have ranged from borderline usefulness to complete ineffectiveness.

Various types of dandruff preparations are discussed in the following question and answer.

DANDRUFF PREPARATIONS

How effective are the various preparations advertised for control of simple dandruff?

Any good shampoo can provide some control over dandruff flaking. As often as the shampoo is used, the scalp is cleansed and itching and flaking subside. Too often, however, these symptoms return in just a few days. So unless the hair is washed every 2 or 3 days, conventional shampoos are usually not a satisfactory answer. Also, frequent shampooing has a drying effect that may cause flaking.

Some medicated products can be more effective than conventional shampoos. They seem to repress the return of more noticeable dandruff symptoms for a longer period of time—5 to 7 days, instead of 2 to 4—and once-a-week washing (which is the custom for most people) is often sufficient to maintain good control.

A doctor may also advise the use of one of several prescription treatments for seborrheic dermatitis, the aggravated form of dandruff. Some of these prescription remedies are also effective when used regularly as preventives. A brand-name guide to antidandruff products is provided at the end of this chapter.

SOAP AND DANDRUFF

Is it true that touching your hairline with soapy hands while washing your face can cause dandruff?

There is no scientific basis for this statement. Shampooing, using soap and water, is recommended for the control of dandruff. Of course, if all the soap is not rinsed off, it may leave a cosmetically undesirable residue that might be confused with dandruff.

HAIR SPRAY AND DANDRUFF

Can hair spray cause dandruff? When I comb my hair after using a spray, there is a great deal of flaking.

Hair sprays have not been incriminated as a cause of dandruff. However, the person using hair spray may already have dandruff. Most hair sprays contain polymers of various types. These produce a film on the hair shaft that sets the hair in the desired position. When the user brushes or combs her hair vigorously, especially after repeated application of hair spray, the film flakes and is shed from the hair shaft, giving the appearance of dandruff.

This flaking is particularly common if the hair-spray container has been held too close to the hair, producing a local heavy concentration rather than a thin film. When the hair is vigorously brushed or combed, this "pool" of excess spray polymer will flake off.

SUMMER HAIR PROBLEMS

In the summertime my hair becomes dry, brittle and discolored. What causes this, and how can it be prevented? What can be done for hair already damaged?

Overexposure to the sun is a common cause of the condition you describe. The easiest way to prevent further difficulty is to avoid excessive exposure to the sun and protect your hair with a scarf or wide-brimmed hat. Some hair sprays contain sunscreens to protect hair in the same way that suntan preparations protect skin from the sun's burning rays, but such protection is probably minimal. Fortunately, the damage is limited to the hair shaft, and the root that controls hair growth is not affected.

Another common cause of dry hair in summer is bathing in saltwater or in chlorinated pools. Always rinse your hair, or even shampoo, after swimming to avoid the damaging effects of chlorinated and salty water.

If your hair is already brittle and dry, gentle brushing with a soft, natural-bristle brush, applications of any oily pomade or hair groom, and less frequent shampooing with a mild shampoo will be helpful. Time alone may cure many hair problems associated with excessive exposure to sun and water during the summer.

Dyeing your hair to cover the streaked portions may not solve the problem, because damaged hair reacts differently to hair coloring agents than does normal hair. When the discoloration is minimal, a water-soluble temporary rinse can help. If you don't like the result, the rinse can be removed with shampoo.

If you need a permanent, a brand made especially for dry, damaged hair is best. Under all circumstances follow the directions carefully.

SINGEING FOR SPLIT ENDS

I've been told that if I have split ends, my hair won't grow. I've also heard that cutting split ends doesn't get rid of them, but that they should be singed. Is this true?
There is no cause for concern when the ends of healthy hair split. Split ends are caused by separation of individual cell layers of the hair. If you are concerned about the cosmetic appearance of your hair, it is necessary to cut off only the section that is split.

The notion that singeing is preferred to cutting is based on the erroneous belief of the past that the entire hair is constantly nourished by a lifegiving fluid that flows through a hollow canal in the hair shaft. It was believed that cutting would open the end of this canal and the nourishing fluid would be lost, causing the hair to die. People also thought that singeing would weld the end into a closed point that would act as a stopper to the vial of lifegiving fluid. In fact, no hollow canal or nourishing fluid exists in the shaft of a human hair; furthermore, the root is the only living portion of a hair. The visible portion (the shaft) is a nonliving structure that cannot "regrow," and there is no scientific value in singeing hair. In fact, singeing may further damage your hair.

WHAT TO DO ABOUT SPLIT ENDS

How can I avoid getting split ends and get rid of the ones I have now?

The only way to get rid of split ends is to cut them off. To avoid getting split ends, don't abuse your hair. If you use an electric hair dryer, set it on medium instead of high. If you prefer electric curlers, don't use them more than two or three times a week (preferably less often). Avoid electric curlers with pointed teeth—they tangle hair. Use smooth-surfaced or foam rollers instead of brush rollers, and a natural bristle or nylon brush with smooth-edged instead of rough-edged bristles. Brush out teasing and tangles starting at the ends of your hair, and don't overtease to begin with.

Conditioners help damaged hair look better and be more manageable, but they can't rejoin split ends or eliminate the problem as some advertisements imply. Split ends occur when the individual cell layers of the hair shaft separate. Protein conditioners coat the hair shaft and may temporarily hold the ends together, but once the "glue" dries out, the split ends reappear. If the outer layer of the hair has been chipped or cracked by physical or chemical abuse (excessive heat, bleaching, permanent waves), the conditioner smoothes and fills in the roughened, uneven surface, making the hair feel smooth and not as dry. But it can't revitalize or change hair permanently, because the hair shaft (the hair above the surface of the scalp) is composed of dead tissue. The longer the hair, the older it is, and the more it has been subjected to abuse. People with short hair are less troubled with split ends than those who have longer hair. But long or short, the better the care, the healthier the hair.

OILY HAIR

I have extremely oily hair that must be shampooed every 2 or 3 days. Can you recommend something to reduce the oiliness?

Shampooing more often with a carefully selected shampoo will help to keep the amount of oil at a minimum. However, external treatments and preparations cannot stop oil from reaching the surface of your hair and scalp; they simply remove oil that has accumulated. Some do this more efficiently than others. A short haircut will make frequent shampooing easier and reduce you hair's ability to accumulate oil.

One method that will enhance the oil-removing effects of shampoo is to wash, rinse, and wash again, leaving the shampoo on your scalp for 5 minutes before rinsing thoroughly.

Commercial shampoos vary considerably as to the amount of oil and soil that they will remove. Some have high detergent or drying characteristics, while others are designed to remove smaller amounts of oil. If commercial shampoos prove unsatisfactory, medicated shampoos and scalp preparations that reduce scalp oiliness are available. These are best prescribed by a physician.

TURNING GRAY OVERNIGHT

Is it true that hair can suddenly turn gray overnight?

Hair turning gray overnight is mentioned in many medical publications as well as in folklore. However, a fully documented, completely convincing report has never appeared in the scientific literature. Scientific knowledge about hair color and growth indicates that such a phenomenon would be impossible, unless some material could be formed that penetrated into the hair shaft and bleached or carried away the pigment. No such material has ever been demonstrated.

Hair color results from the depositing of color pigments along the inside of the hair shaft. These pigments are produced by cells near the root and deposited in the hair as it forms. When hair turns gray or white, pigment cells become inactive and future hairs will be unpigmented, or gray. However, the pigmented hairs already present are not affected.

In ordinary graying, which is a normal part of aging, the process usually is slow but progressive. On rare occasions graying can result from disease or some other condition. In these instances the onset of graying may be sudden, with pigment cells in most or all hair follicles ceasing production at the same time. As a new hair grows in, it will be gray, but the part that already is pigmented will not change color. All new hairs will be unpigmented (gray), making the change much more evident.

Turning gray overnight is possible when a person already has both pigmented hairs and gray hairs and all of the pigmented hairs are shed at once, leaving only the gray hairs. This may occur in the unusual form of baldness called alopecia areata. Or all the pigmented hairs may be shed within a short period of time, making it more obvious that the color of scalp hair has changed, though without any sudden change in the color of individual hairs.

REPIGMENTATION OF GRAY HAIR

Is it possible for gray hair to return to its original color?
Senile graying of the hair, a normal part of aging, is an irreversible process. We are not aware of any well-documented case in which hair color returned after loss of color associated with aging.

If hair graying results from disease, the color may be restored either temporarily or permanently when the patient recovers. In such cases, pigmented hair begins to grow out from the roots, so individual hairs may be white at the tip while the portion nearest the roots is repigmented. Or hairs may have alternate bands of more and less pigment as the pigment-forming capacity waxes and wanes with the severity of the disease. However, color will not be restored to that part of the hair already formed; it will remain gray.

Hair may gray as a result of endocrine gland disorders; injury or disease of the nervous system; physical and mental shock; and severe illnesses such as typhus, malaria, and influenza. If and when hair grows back following alopecia areata, the hairs are initially white or gray; however, color is usually restored in later growth. (Alopecia areata is discussed in the previous chapter on hair loss.)

HAZARDS OF TEASING HAIR

Are hair-styling methods such as roughing, teasing, and back-combing harmful or damaging to my hair, and if so, to what extent?

Roughing, back-combing, and teasing hair are basically identical techniques. They give added body to hair styles and do not damage hair if performed properly and if your hair is in good condition. However, they should be performed gently and not too often in order to minimize roughening and tangling, especially if your hair is dry and brittle or breaks easily. Excessive tension on hair during teasing may produce temporary hair loss, such as sometimes results from wearing tight ponytails and braids. If you like a style that requires teasing, it would be wise to have it done properly by an expert rather than attempting to do it yourself.

Teasing tends to tangle hair badly; tangled hair is difficult to comb and may break more often. Brushing is actually more effective than combing and is easier on your hair. To remove tangling, begin combing or brushing at the ends, working toward the scalp and removing the tangles gently.

TREATMENT FOR DAMAGED HAIR

Do preparations and treatments that claim to help damaged hair actually affect the structure of hair and make it stronger?

Methods that claim to improve the condition of damaged hair are limited mainly to improving the luster and finish of hair fibers. They include hot oil applications, oil shampoos, and treatment with creams containing emollients such as lanolin, cholesterol, and fatty alcohols. Hair rinses and conditioners based on protein ingredients or fiber softeners help improve the appearance of hair and make it more manageable. Such treatments do nothing to increase the tensile strength and elasticity of weakened, damaged hair fibers, but the oily coating may make the hair less brittle.

Hair damage most commonly occurs from mechanical teasing and from chemical treatments such as excessive bleaching, waving, or straightening. Such procedures should be stopped when damage is noticed. As new, undamaged hair grows out, the damaged hair should be cut off.

THE HAIRCUT MYTH

My hairdresser tells me to get my long hair cut often because it'll grow faster. This doesn't make sense to me, but considering how much he gets for each trim it probably makes a lot of sense to him. Is he right?

Cutting hair does not make it grow faster, but a good trim can make a head of hair look thicker simply because the scraggly ends are eliminated. Each hair grows at its own pace, so within a few weeks of a haircut the ends become scraggly and uneven. How often it's cut or how much is cut off doesn't affect the growth cycle at all. Your hairdresser's advice is good; it's just the reasoning that's wrong. But you'd probably still do all right to submit to the scissors on a regular basis, especially if you have long hair.

LONG HAIR

How can I make my hair grow longer? It's always been short and nothing I do seems to change that.

Unfortunately, once your hair has grown to its full length, there is nothing you can do to make it grow longer. Scalp hairs usually grow for 2 to 6 years at about one-half inch per month. After a scalp hair stops growing, it goes into a resting phase of several months; then it falls out and a new hair begins to grow. Each hair has its own growth cycle so that at any given time approximately 85 percent are in the growing phase and 15 percent in the resting phase. The length of the growing phase, which depends on your genetic makeup, determines the final length your hair will reach—assuming it has never been cut. If your hair has a 2-year growing period, for example, the most you can hope for are 12-inch tresses.

To find out if this is the cause of your "short" hair, check the ends. The tips of normally growing, undamaged and uncut hair come to very fine points. (You might find you have split or frayed hair, but if the original tip is there your hair is growing as long as your genes allow it.) However, if the ends of your hair are sharply cut, blunt or jagged, it means that the shafts have been cut or broken and that your hair is not growing to its normal length. The culprit could be excessive brushing with hard, nylon brushes; rough teasing; excessive heat from electric rollers and hair driers; exposure to sunlight or chlorinated or salt water; too much shampooing, overbleaching, straightening, or other such treatments. If your hair is short because of mishandling, proper care will help give you greater length.

In rare cases, short hair results from a medical problem (malnutrition, severe hormonal imbalance, or improper thyroid functioning). But if you're feeling well and have no specific complaints, this probably isn't your problem.

You may want to experiment with a wig or fall as a means of achieving a long hair style. Well-fitting synthetic fiber wigs and falls are available in a variety of long styles and colors at modest prices. With a little practice, you should be able to comb and style your hairpiece to look very natural. Anchoring the wig or fall with bobby pins will help to keep it in place. And since wigs are so popular, no one will know whether you are wearing a wig from necessity or by choice.

HEAT DAMAGE TO HAIR

To what temperatures can hair be exposed from driers, hot combs, curling irons and heated rollers without becoming damaged?

The extent to which hair will assume new shapes and the duration over which it will preserve these shapes depends on the treatment temperature. Hair becomes increasingly plastic, and its softness is not quite uniform as the temperature is raised. Significant alterations occur at approximately 140° to 250°F. Large-scale, irreversible damage to hair occurs even with a short exposure only above 300°F. This damage involves both the chemical composition of the hair and its physical structure. Of the group of electrical appliances mentioned above, only heated metal combs—used primarily for straightening kinky hair—operate at temperatures approaching or even slightly exceeding this danger zone. Repeated exposure to these temperatures can weaken the hair so much that temporary hair loss can result due to excessive breakage. Normal hair growth may require many months to overcome this defect.

All other classes of heated hair appliances from reputable manufacturers, bearing the UL seal of approval, work at significantly lower temperatures than heated metal combs. Under recommended conditions they cause no changes in the chemical structure of the hair, and their physical effects are minimal, even with frequent use.

Unexpected thermal damage to hair results mostly from the use of defective appliances. Excessive physical damage to hair from the use of heated appliances is due mostly to their improper use. At elevated temperatures, hair in its softened state is less able to resist physical abuse in the form of stretching, clipping, etc., than at room temperature. (Curling irons and heated curlers are discussed in Chapter 8, "Miscellaneous Hair Products." Hot comb straightening is discussed in Chapter 7, "Hair Waving and Straightening.")

CRADLE CAP

What can be done for "cradle cap" in babies?
Cradle cap is a mixture of grease and scales that piles up on the crown of an infant's head to form a coating resembling a cap. The exact cause is not known, but it may result from neglect during bathing for fear of injuring the "soft spot."

Cradle cap is not serious unless secondary infection occurs beneath the heavy crusts and scales. Temporary hair loss may be seen when hairs are dislodged by the crust. Frequent gentle shampooing often alleviates cradle cap. If it does not, consult your physician.

OIL TREATMENTS FOR DRY HAIR

Will hot oil treatments help dry hair and scalp?
Hot oil treatments by competent beauticians will relieve excessively dry hair and scaling scalp to some degree temporarily. If the hair is too dry and brittle due to external damage, it will not regain its natural sheen and pliability until new hair grows out, and this may take many months. If excessive dryness is due to either hereditary or acquired disease of the oil glands and hair follicles, hot oil treatments will not be effective. A physician's treatment will be required.

CURE FOR DRAB HAIR

How can I add luster to dull, drab hair?
Dull, drab hair is most often caused by excessive dryness, oiliness, and other damage to hair resulting from overexposure to

the sun or excessive or improper use of hair waving, straightening, bleaching, or coloring preparations. Too much hair spray or wave set, or failure to remove all the soap from your hair when shampooing, can produce a dull film. Sometimes dull, drab hair is associated with illnesses, internal disorders, or dietary deficiencies.

Shampoos specially formulated for dry hair, followed by the application of a creme rinse or conditioner, help to counteract dryness and add luster. Hot oil treatments by a competent beautician provide temporary help to dry, damaged hair. If hair damage has resulted from waving, straightening, or coloring, such harmful procedures should be stopped to allow new, undamaged hair to grow out.

If the problem is caused by excessive oiliness, more frequent shampooing—every day if necessary—may solve the problem. Use a shampoo specially formulated for oily hair. To enhance the oil-removing effect of the shampoo, wash, rinse, and wash again, leaving the preparation on your scalp for five minutes before rinsing thoroughly.

A short hair style makes frequent shampooing easier and minimizes the accumulation of oil.

CARE OF FINE HAIR

What kind of care is recommended for fine, thin hair?
No treatment will make fine hair thicker, since this is usually an inherited characteristic. But treatments are available to make fine hair more manageable. A body permanent specially designed for fine hair adds body and helps hair sets last longer. Some people find that using a bleach or tint makes hair more manageable, but the long-term damaging effect of bleaching tends to rule out this treatment. Conditioners containing ingredients such as proteins and oils deposit a film on the hair that adds body temporarily and may make it seem thicker.

In rare instances fine, sparse, or dry hair is not an inherited characteristic but is secondary to some internal disturbance affecting the growth of the skin, hair and nails. For example, fine, sparse hair in infants or young children may be associated with problems such as inborn errors of metabolism. In such cases a physician should be consulted to determine the cause and to treat the condition.

FREQUENCY OF SHAMPOOING

I have oily hair and I like to wash it every day. My girl-friend told me that this is bad and will make my hair fall out. How often can I wash it without losing it?

Hair can and should be shampooed as often as necessary to keep it clean and the scalp comfortable. Whenever hair becomes dull, lacks luster, and loses its set, it is probably time to shampoo.

Usually, once a week is adequate, but some people—most often those with oily hair like yours—may need to shampoo as often as every day. Your girlfriend is misinformed; there is no truth to the notion that frequent washing will cause hair loss.

However, if you seem to be losing more than the normal amount of hair (everybody loses from forty to sixty hairs a day regularly, and new hairs grow in to replace the lost ones), it could be because you are overly vigorous in your shampooing or hair drying—that is, you are breaking your hair by rubbing it too hard with the towel.

HAIR AND SCALP CARE

What do you suggest for proper care of the hair and scalp?

Good grooming for everyone has many aspects, and care of the hair and scalp is an important one. Good care is not complicated. It requires only a few ingredients: regular shampooing, a comb and brush, and a timely trip to the barbershop or beauty parlor.

Hair should be shampooed as often as needed. Once a week is usually recommended, but hair can be washed more often with perfect safety. People with oily hair and those exposed to city dirt or unusually active physical exertion may find it desirable to shampoo twice or perhaps even three times a week. Some shampoo daily.

Before shampooing your hair, brush it free of all tangles (this also removes surface dirt). Next, wet your hair thoroughly and use plenty of lather. Massage your scalp, using fingertips rather than nails to avoid scratches. Rinse your hair very carefully, being sure to remove all traces of suds. Follow with a creme rinse or conditioner if desired.

Blot your hair dry to prevent tangles. Avoid brisk rubbing. Comb wet hair with a wide-toothed comb; don't brush it. If you use a dryer, regulate it carefully to avoid overheating, which will make your hair dry, brittle and easy to damage with a comb or brush.

Daily brushing supplements regular shampoos. Brushing helps to keep your hair and scalp clean by loosening and removing dust, grime, hair spray residue, and dead cells. The best way to brush is from the roots, stroking toward the ends. Brushing is more gentle than combing for removing snarls and tangles from hair and adds luster. Brush whenever you want your hair to look its best in the morning, in the evening, or in between. But don't brush your hair excessively (forget about 100 strokes a day)—and don't brush your scalp too vigorously or it may become irritated. Use a soft brush and keep both brush and comb clean by washing them frequently in warm, soapy water.

NYLON VS. NATURAL BRISTLE BRUSHES AND EXCESSIVE BRUSHING

Should I brush my hair 100 strokes a day to keep it healthy? Is it true that nylon brushes are more damaging to the hair than natural bristle brushes?

Forget about the old directive to "brush your hair 100 strokes a day." Brushing by itself won't make your hair healthier—and may even damage it.

Excessive brushing, massaging, and other kinds of manipulation can irritate your scalp and contribute to hair breakage and split ends. It can also cause premature loss of hairs that are in the resting stage of the growth cycle and not firmly attached in the hair follicle. This is especially true if your hair is already damaged or "unhealthy"—a time when, unfortunately, people start overmanipulating hair on the theory that such measures are helpful.

Hair should be brushed or combed no more than is necessary to keep it neat and attractive. As a rule, twenty or thirty strokes are more than enough to distribute oil along the hair shafts, remove tangles, and whisk away loose dirt, dead cells, and hair spray residue that may be present.

The type of brush is not too important as long as brushing is not excessive. Some nylon "bristle" brushes are considered potentially more damaging to hair than natural bristle brushes because of the shape of the "bristle" tips.

Animal bristles used for natural bristle brushes, most often boar hairs, have tapered tips as part of their normal structure. The cut edges of nylon filaments used for brush bristles are rough and jagged and can irritate the scalp and contribute to hair breakage and split ends unless they are polished or rounded off.

Look closely to determine whether the tips of nylon bristles have been rounded off. As a rule, inexpensive nylon brushes are more apt to have rough-edged bristles, since smoothing the tips adds to manufacturing costs.

AGE AND GRAY HAIR

Is it possible for a sixty-two-year-old man to retain his natural hair color without any graying? An acquaintance of mine who has reached this age has no gray hair, but claims he does not dye his hair.

Graying hair is a normal part of aging, and most people develop noticeable gray hairs by the middle forties. A few lucky people make it to fifty without gray or white hairs, and it is not uncommon to see the change postponed until the middle fifties or even later.

It is unusual for persons past seventy years of age not to have at least some gray hairs. Gray hair usually begins at the temples and gradually extends to the rest of the hair on the head; generally blonds begin to gray before brunettes.

It is possible that your friend still retains his natural hair color. If he dyes it, a close inspection of hair growth at the temples and close to the scalp should show gray hair. It is also likely that he has at least a few scattered gray hairs, even though they aren't noticeable.

GREEN HAIR

Why does my blond hair develop a green discoloration when I swim in chlorinated swimming pools in the summer? What can I do to prevent this, and to remove discoloration already present?

Products called algicides, which are added to swimming pools to retard the growth of algae, are primarily responsible for the greenish discoloration of blond hair. These algicides often contain copper compounds that interact with chlorine in the water to produce a greenish deposit on the hair. Wearing a bathing cap will help to prevent discoloration.

We are not aware of any simple home remedy for removing the greenish discoloration, but we understand that beauty salons can provide various treatments to conceal or remove it. These treatments require careful and expert use; we therefore suggest that you consult a beautician about removing any discoloration already present in your hair.

BRAND-NAME GUIDE TO ANTIDANDRUFF PRODUCTS*

	Sulfur	Tar	Salicylic Acid	Zinc Pyrithione	Selenium Sulfide	Antibacterial Agents	Quaternary Ammonium Salts
SHAMPOOS							
Breck One				•			
Double Danderine							•
Enden Cream and Lotion	•						
Fostex	•		•				
Head and Shoulders				•			
Ionil							•
Meted/Meted 2	•		•				
Pentrax		•					
Rezamid	•		•				
Sebb						•	
Sebulex	•		•				
Sebutone	•	•	•				
Selsun Blue					•		
Zetar		•	•			•	
SHAMPOO TREATMENTS *Prescription Only*							
Selsun					•		
POST-SHAMPOO TREATMENTS *Over-the-Counter*							
Dandricide							•
Rinse Away							•
Scadan							•
HAIRDRESSINGS							
Sebucare				•			
Top Brass						•	
ZP-11					•		

*This guide lists popular brands in national distribution but makes no attempt to list all on the market.

DAILY SWIMMING AND ~~EXCESSIVE~~ TANGLING OF HAIR

I swim every day, most~~ly laps~~. I find that my scalp hair, especially in the back, ~~ge~~ts tangled and hard to comb. What causes this problem and is there a remedy?

Daily swimming, especially in a chlorinated pool, may contribute to hair problems, including tangling. Chlorinated water dries hair, and daily shampooing may also contribute to hair problems, especially when combined with exposure to chlorinated water. Both factors decrease the hair's normal protective oily film. Finally, wet hair tangles easily and vigorous combing may result in hair breakage.

To minimize the adverse effects of daily swimming and shampooing, a hair care program that includes the following procedures may be helpful:

Use a mild shampoo formulated for dry or damaged hair, soaping only once to minimize the removal of oil.

Apply a creme rinse or some other postshampoo conditioner to your hair following shampooing. These preparations deposit a light film on the hair to minimize tangling, aid combing, and counteract dryness and static electricity that causes "fly-away" hair.

Dry your hair by wrapping it in a towel and gently patting or squeezing out excess water. Do not rub your hair vigorously; it contributes to tangling and breakage. Gently comb wet hair with a wide and blunt-toothed comb. Don't try to brush wet hair. A short, simple hair style requires less care to look attractive, and short hair has less tendency to tangle.

Wear a swimming cap that keeps your hair as dry as possible. While no cap keeps hair completely dry if you dive or swim vigorously, some caps do a better job than others.

Part III
SKIN

13

Acne—Blemishes

THE WHY OF ACNE

*What causes acne? I understand that there is no cure. I
would like to know, however, what treatments are helpful.*
Acne is a very common skin condition afflicting most people
in varying degrees and for varying periods, especially during
the teen years. It consists of blackheads, whiteheads, pustules,
and sometimes deeper boil-like blemishes. Acne is not a single
disease; there are several varieties, each with its own characteristics.

Acne most commonly occurs on the face, but often also
appears on the back, chest, shoulders, and neck. In severe
cases it may be widespread. Acne is not a medically serious
disease, but it is disfiguring at a time when young people are
most sensitive about their appearance. Furthermore, it can
lead to serious and permanent scarring.

Acne occurs at the time of adolescence when endocrine
gland activity increases. These glands secrete hormones that
contribute to many of our characteristics (for instance, secondary sex characteristics), change children into adults, and affect
various parts of the body including the sebaceous (oil) glands
of the skin.

At adolescence the sebaceous glands enlarge and become
active. This enlargement and the excess of oily material
(sebum) that the sebaceous glands produce are the essential

features of acne. While most of the oil produced by the glands reaches the surface, some may be dammed back in the ducts of the large oil glands and produce blackheads and whiteheads. These may eventually break through the walls of the ducts to produce pimples and boil-like lesions of acne. (See "Antibiotics for Acne" elsewhere in this chapter for additional information on formation of acne lesions.)

The fact that acne is common does not mean that nothing can be done for it. Waiting to "outgrow" acne can be a serious mistake. While there is no instant and permanent cure for acne, it can be treated and controlled. Supervision by a physician will help ensure minimal skin involvement and scarring. (See the following answer for details about treatment.)

CONTROLLING ACNE

What can I do to get rid of the pimples on my face? They make me very self-conscious. I am fourteen years old and watch what I eat. I've tried different kinds of preparations from the drugstore, but they don't help much.

Acne is a problem common to many young people in your age group. It usually begins with the onset of puberty (eleven to thirteen years) and disappears gradually in the early twenties. This period varies, however, with each individual.

Acne cannot be prevented or cured at present, but proper treatment will control or minimize it and lessen the likelihood of pitting and scarring.

Acne is not caused by dirt, but, since it is most often associated with oily skin, washing your face with soap and hot water three or four times each day helps to control the oiliness. Some physicians advise using soap that contains an antiseptic to decrease bacteria on the skin surface. Frequent shampooing is also important because hair is often excessively oily.

Lotions and creams available at drugstores may help in treating acne; however, many cause too much dryness if used excessively. If you use these products, follow the manufacturer's instructions carefully. If your skin becomes irritated, use them less often or stop entirely. For covering blemishes, medicated preparations have been formulated that match skin color. Ordinary makeup should not be used regularly; use nonoily cosmetics instead and remove them thoroughly at bedtime.

If acne persists even when you follow such a routine, see a physician. A great deal more can be done to help you, and seeking medical care may prevent permanent damage. After examining you, the physician can determine the important aspects of your treatment. Do not assume that medicine and methods prescribed for a friend will necessarily be good for you.

Methods and medications for treating acne vary from one physician to another, and treatment also varies with the needs of the individual patient. Even though treatment often involves nothing more than simple local skin care, you must understand that control of acne is a long-term, continuing process. Follow the instructions of your physician faithfully and regularly. Other aspects of acne treatments are discussed in the following questions and answers.

NO FAST "CURE" FOR ACNE

I have tried just about everything on the market for my acne, but nothing has helped. Please tell me what I can do to get rid of my blemishes.

First, you must realize that there is no simple or short-term treatment for acne. This skin disorder must be viewed as a chronic disease of the teen years that can be adequately controlled but not cured. Acne is stubborn and unpredictable, and its treatment varies in different individuals. Mild cases may be helped in varying degrees by over-the-counter (OTC) medications (as discussed elsewhere in this chapter), but many cases require treatment by a physician.

If you have tried self-treatment without success, consult

a physician. In prescribing medications, the physician can adjust the dosage and proportion of ingredients to meet your specific needs, and can prescribe topical and internal medications, such as antibiotics, that are available only on prescription. These medications may be combined with other treatment methods such as cryosurgery or use of a sunlamp. While these treatments will not "cure" your acne, they will help to minimize the severity of the lesions and the scarring that often follows acne, as well as improve your cosmetic appearance.

CYSTIC ACNE

Our sixteen-year-old son has cystic acne. This condition remains severe, even though he is being treated by a dermatologist. We would appreciate any information you can give us on this type of acne.

Several types of acne are often called cystic acne. Therefore it is not possible to be specific in answering your question. Patients with cystic acne, in general, represent the most challenging problem in the therapy of acne. This type of acne can lead to considerable scarring, so it is important that the patient be under the care of a dermatologist. Although the disease will eventually clear by itself, failure to get treatment while awaiting spontaneous cure may lead to increased scarring.

It should be understood that this type of acne is very difficult to treat even under close medical supervision, with drugs and surgery available. As with many chronic conditions, the patient must persist in therapy. Some scarring may be unavoidable.

ACNE IN ADULTS

I'm thirty-one years old and have had acne since I was a teenager. I've consulted physicians and used many medications. Are any new, successful treatments available? Will I have acne forever?

Acne is a condition that can be controlled, not cured. This is true no matter how old the patient is. Although acne disappears of its own accord in most patients by about age twenty, it unfortunately persists in a small percentage of cases well into adulthood. A few women continue to have acne until menopause; in a very small percentage of persistent cases, an endocrine or other abnormality may be present. A thorough medical evaluation may be of value.

Contraceptive pills control the problem for a number of women as well as girls who have attained full growth. Results usually appear 2 or 3 months after the drug has been started. Estrogenic substances may be helpful, too. Orally administered antibiotics have been a great aid in controlling the inflammatory and infectious aspects of the problem. When effective, these drugs must be continued under the supervision of a physician.

Adequate skin care (blackhead removal, drainage of cysts, ultraviolet exposure, drying and peeling preparations), as well as general dietary and health care, should be continued.

BLACKHEADS

I have oily skin and wash with a special soap, but I still have blackheads, especially on my nose. What can I do?
First of all, blackheads are not caused by dirt or bacteria, so special soaps and excessive scrubbing won't get rid of them. Blackheads form when pores or ducts on the skin are blocked, and oil produced by the glands can't reach the skin surface. The oil turns black because of oxidation and the presence of certain particles of skin pigment (melanin). Areas most apt to develop blackheads are the nose, forehead, and chin, which have large, active oil glands. There is no cure for blackheads, but here are some tips that will help you control them.

Wash frequently with soap and water. This dries the skin and causes mild peeling, which helps eliminate plug formation. Remember, special soaps are not necessary, and abrasive cleansers and complexion brushes may irritate your skin and have no special cleansing powers.

During the day, remove excess oil with an astringent. Take care not to irritate your skin with excessive use, and avoid creams and oily cosmetics. If you use a cream to remove makeup, follow up with a thorough soap and water cleansing.

You may want to try one of the drying and peeling lotions available, but don't go overboard, and cut back if you notice any redness or irritation. Natural and artificial sunlight also induce dryness and peeling, but overexposure and sunburn should be avoided.

Unless you know the proper technique for squeezing blackheads—don't. You'll only injure the surrounding skin and help spread the oily material, causing more problems. Your doctor can show you the proper way to remove blackheads and will advise you how often it should be done—usually once a week or every 2 weeks is sufficient. If you have any questions about commercial blackhead extractors or other treatments, check with your doctor. Blackheads are a stage of acne and deserve proper treatment.

SUN'S EFFECT ON ACNE

My skin blemishes seem to clear up during the summer months. Does the sun have a beneficial effect?
Yes, cautious initial sun exposure increased slowly allows the skin to peel and improves some cases of acne. An ultraviolet bulb or sunlamp will produce similar results, but special precautions must be taken to avoid a burn.

Seek your physician's advice regarding treatment for your case. Some people respond best to sunlight only when local medications are used at the same time. Other cases may even be made worse by exposure to the sun.

You should also know that overexposure to sunlight results in some undesirable skin changes such as premature aging and skin cancer. These changes are discussed in Chapter 20, "Sunlight and the Skin."

SEX, SLEEP, AND ACNE

Is it true that sexual activity and lack of sleep have a bad influence on acne?

Many old wives' tales are associated with acne, and one of the most common is the notion that sex and acne are somehow related. Neither sexual activity nor sexual inactivity has any effect at all on acne, although it is true that sex hormones play a role in acne.

Years ago many physicians thought that fatigue and exhaustion aggravated acne, and therefore recommended that acne patients get plenty of sleep. Now most authorities, while in favor of adequate sleep and general good health, do not consider sleep an important factor in controlling acne.

DIET AND ACNE

What foods should I avoid to help clear up my acne? I have been told that chocolate, soft drinks, and fatty, fried foods are especially bad for acne.

Diet does not play a major role in acne, and following the diet will not by itself clear acne, although some foods may aggravate acne in some people. A number of foods that in the past have been blamed for aggravating acne now, after further study, appear to be relatively blameless. Several studies indicate that even large amounts of chocolate may have little effect on the course of acne in most people, although more controlled studies are needed to clarify this point. Large amounts of fat in the diet also appear blameless.

On the other hand, most physicians agree that iodides and bromides can cause skin eruptions that look like acne. Excessive intakes should probably be curtailed during acne treatment. Iodides occur in appreciable amounts in iodized salt, saltwater fish, and shellfish. Certain drugs such as cough medicines, sedatives, cold medications, and multivitamin mineral combinations may contain iodides or bromides. Iodides should not be completely eliminated from the diet, however, or goiters may develop.

If it seems to you that certain foods, whether chocolate, soft drinks, dairy products, or fried foods, aggravate your acne, try dropping the apparent offender from your diet and observe your skin's reactions. After a few weeks, reintroduce the food and again observe the effect. If your acne flares up, try to avoid that food.

"PIMPLES" AND MENSTRUATION

My skin breaks out at the time of my menstrual period. What treatment is advised?

A number of dermatologic diseases are aggravated at times in the menstrual cycle of some women, including the breakout of "pimples" (acne). The exact reason for these breakouts is not known, although they are probably related in some way to the hormones secreted by the ovaries.

Active local treatment of the skin, internal treatment with antibiotics, restriction of salt intake, medically supervised therapy to reduce water retention just before menstruation, or possibly therapy with hormones may be required to control these breakouts. Treatment must be individualized for each patient by her physician, and recurrence can usually be prevented through a suitable treatment schedule.

PIMPLES AND COSMETICS

Every once in a while I break out in pimples. Should I stop using cosmetics at such times?

Powders and oily cosmetic bases may aggravate your skin condition. Nonoily preparations are preferable, but should be thoroughly removed at bedtime. Medicated preparations are available for masking blemishes temporarily, with tints added to match natural skin color.

HAIR STYLES AND ACNE

Can a hair style with bangs or hanging hair make my acne worse?

Some teenagers wear their hair in long hair styles that fall over the forehead and face in order to conceal acne; others wear their hair this way because the style is popular. Regardless of the reason for such hair styles, acne can be made worse by overhanging hair. Although there is disagreement on why over-hanging hair may aggravate acne, most dermatologists feel that there is a relationship; therefore patients with acne are advised to keep their hair off the face, at least when they are not appearing in public.

Washing the skin often is an important part of acne treatment, and a young man or girl with long hanging hair may tend to slight the covered skin areas in cleansing and in applying medications. Hair also shields the face from the sun's rays, which generally are helpful for acne. These may be reasons why the disease flares up on the forehead under the hair.

SHAVING AND ACNE

What is the best method of shaving when you have acne?

No one method has proved superior. Some young men prefer blade razors; others find electric razors more helpful. The best advice is to use the shaving method that is least irritating and most comfortable for you. In rare cases, the only approach is to grow a beard.

One consultant suggested the following tips to the acne sufferer. (1) Shave with the grain and as seldom as possible (maybe once or twice a week); (2) if you prefer a wet shave, use a new blade each time; (3) soften your beard by washing carefully with plenty of soap and hot water; (4) leave lather or shaving cream on for at least a minute before you start to shave; (5) after shaving, rinse with hot water, then cold water —and you may apply an astringent antiseptic lotion (if not irritating).

FACIAL SAUNAS FOR ACNE

How safe and effective are facial saunas for treating acne? Facial sauna devices have been promoted for the treatment of acne, but there is no evidence that they provide special benefits; physicians have seen some cases in which acne was worsened by exposure to saunas.

Electrical units that use the term "sauna" are designed to heat water, releasing steam vapor to which the face is then exposed. Actually, "facial steam baths" might be a more appropriate name for these devices, since true sauna baths use dry rather than moist air; the humidity of true saunas rarely rises above 15 percent.

Advertisers claim that these devices cause the skin to perspire, cleansing it "deep-down." But sweating will not flush out pores, nor is steaming enough to cleanse the face. In some cases excessive sweating aggravates acne. The combination of steam and sweating when used excessively may produce a form of acne known as tropical acne.

Soap-and-water cleansing is still required after a "sauna" treatment, and it is quite likely that thorough soap-and-water cleansing alone is equally, if not more, effective in this regard. Claims by any chemical or mechanical product for "super-cleansing" or "deep-down cleansing" should be viewed with skepticism, since cleansing does not go below the surface of the skin.

Remember that it is not possible to open and close pores, despite the popular impression that this is true. Also remember that acne blemishes are not caused by dirt. The reason frequent washing is recommended in the treatment of acne is that washing causes increased dryness and peeling of the skin, which are desirable in most cases. For details see previous questions and answers in this section on the cause and control of acne.

Manufacturers of one facial sauna device also claim that steam-vapor treatments make the skin more accessible to penetration by medication. While heat and moisture may facilitate the penetration of certain topical medications, there is no evidence that facial saunas will do this, or that such penetration is desirable in the treatment of acne.

The Federal Food and Drug Administration has seized several sauna devices because of false and misleading claims that the devices were adequate and effective in treating various health problems including acne and skin blemishes.

In most cases proper use of facial saunas will not harm the skin, but don't expect them to cure acne or any other health problem. These devices may temporarily increase circulation to the skin and introduce quite a bit of moisture into the uppermost layers, but whether this helps is doubtful. The effect may be relaxing, as is applying a warm, wet towel to the face, but don't expect more. There is no magic in these devices.

In the past, various hormones have been used to reduce hyperactivity of the sebaceous glands (oil glands of the skin).

HORMONE AND VITAMIN PREPARATIONS FOR ACNE

What are the relative values of hormones and vitamins for treating acne?

Both agents have been used in treating acne. Oral vitamin A has been prescribed, for example, in cases of acne that consist primarily of blackheads. However, authorities do not agree on the efficacy of this treatment. Recently, topical application of tretinoin (vitamin A acid) has relieved some relatively severe cases of acne. At present, there appears to be no rationale for the use of other vitamin preparations.

Since overactive sebaceous glands are an integral part of

the acne process, any agent that decreases this activity will aid in treatment of the disease. Adequate dosages of estrogen, a female hormone, will decrease the size of the sebaceous glands and thus reduce the amount of oily material produced. However, estrogen treatment can be used only in females because the dosage required to treat acne tends to produce feminine characteristics when given to young males.

Many different estrogen preparations are available. Oral contraceptives, which contain estrogen, have also been used for this purpose. However, estrogen preparations must be given under a physician's guidance. Commercially available topical preparations containing estrogenic hormones do not appear to contain enough hormones to be effective.

WASHING AND SPECIAL SOAPS FOR ACNE

If acne is not caused by dirt, why did my doctor tell me to wash my face several times a day? Are special soaps better than plain soap for acne?

While acne is not caused by dirt, most physicians recommend that their acne patients wash several times a day for other reasons. Washing helps to remove oil, dead skin, and surface bacteria and may be of some help in mild acne.

For cleansing the skin, ordinary commercial soaps usually do an adequate job. Special acne soaps containing tar and sulfur, among other ingredients, provide few, if any, additional benefits. Nor are antibacterial soaps generally helpful, since the bacteria associated with acne are below the surface of the skin. In severe cases of acne, however, a physician may recommend using an antibacterial soap to help minimize secondary infections of acne lesions. Some physicians also prefer tincture of green soap to ordinary soap, although it may prove to be drying and irritating.

Abrasive soaps that contain irritating granules are of some value for certain persons, but they can be quite harsh to sensitive skin and therefore should be used with caution. These soaps induce physically the therapeutic inflammation and peeling that antiacne medications cause chemically. It is best to start by using an abrasive soap once a day and then more frequently if your skin can tolerate it. If your skin becomes red, irritated, and peels too much from use of abrasive soap, cut down on frequency of use, using it only occasionally or not at all. If you are using abrasive soap, consult your physician to be sure that its use is properly integrated into your total acne care program.

MEDICATED COSMETICS FOR ACNE

Are medicated cosmetics better for my skin if I have acne? Will they help to cure my pimples?

A number of cosmetic products are promoted to acne-prone teenagers with claims that the products are "medicated" and thus better for the person who has acne or pimples.

In the case of face makeups, the basis for "medicated" claims usually is the incorporation of various antibacterial ingredients into the product. The main function of many of these preparations is camouflage (i.e., hiding blemishes, skin discolorations, and ruddy or sallow coloring, and evening out skin tone), but in their advertising and labeling they promise or appear to promise therapeutic benefits. The use of mild antibacterials with a medicated aroma fortifies the slogan "clean makeup" (what is "dirty makeup"?). In fact, the addition of these ingredients serves no beneficial purpose in helping to clear up blemishes since acne is not an infectious disease. The antibacterial ingredients do help to preserve the product itself from bacterial attack.

Other "medicated" cosmetic products are basically skin fresheners or astringents to which antibacterial or antiseptic ingredients, mild topical analgesics or counterirritants, and/or drying, peeling agents such as resorcinol or salicylic acid may be added. These products are useful in removing excess oil from the skin and promoting dryness and mild peeling—but "non-medicated" preparations will provide the same effects.

If you have acne, avoid heavy, oily cosmetics and don't wear cosmetics all the time. Use them when you need to look your best. Select cosmetics from those formulated for use on oily skin. You may even find that you prefer a "medicated" cosmetic, but don't expect therapeutic effects on acne blemishes. And be sure to remove the makeup at bedtime.

OVER-THE-COUNTER REMEDIES FOR ACNE

What is your opinion of the many nonprescription preparations advertised for treating acne? I don't have a severe acne problem, so I thought I might try some of these products.

Some over-the-counter (OTC) medications may be helpful in treating mild cases of acne, but others are not very helpful at all. Antiacne aids come in a wide variety of forms: creams, cleansers, lotions, soaps, powders, gels, cleansing sticks, scrubs, beauty masques, and medicated towelettes. No single product is ideal for everyone with blemishes. People's skins differ in sensitivity and acne problems differ in magnitude.

Don't waste your money on products such as certain makeup preparations that claim to help acne because they contain "antibacterial" ingredients. Although certain bacteria are the source of enzymes that break down oils into the irritating, acne-producing free fatty acids, these bacteria live beneath the skin's surface, deep in the follicles. They cannot be reached by topical antibacterial agents applied to the surface of the skin.

Ingredients commonly used in OTC remedies that physicians consider of some value in treating acne are sulfur, resorcinol and salicylic acid. (Check the product label for a listing of the active ingredients.) These ingredients cause the skin to peel and, incidentally, produce inflammation and redness. Peeling is considered beneficial, but the products may cause excessive peeling and irritation in some people, especially if applied vigorously or too often. If you want to try one of these products, carefully read and follow the directions supplied with the product. If your skin becomes inflamed and scaly, use the product less frequently or stop using it for a while. Also cut down on your use of soap. If discomfort or scaliness persist, consult a physician.

Premoistened medicated towelettes may be useful for cleansing the skin when washing is inconvenient, as during school or work hours. The towelettes are moistened with solutions containing alcohol or other solvents that remove excess oil from the face. Other ingredients may be added to enhance drying effects and soap may be added for cleansing.

The benefits of special soaps are discussed in the following exchange.

ANTIBIOTICS FOR ACNE

How do antibiotics help acne if it isn't caused by bacteria? My physician prescribed tetracycline for my acne and I've been taking it for several months. While it seems to help, I'm worried that it might be harmful, especially if taken over a long period of time.

Bacteria on the skin's surface do not play a significant role in acne, but bacteria below the surface in the hair follicles do play a role. As stated elsewhere in this chapter, acne is related to the activity of the skin's oil glands. These glands enlarge during adolescence and begin producing large quantities of sebum, an oily mixture of fats and waxes. The oil glands open into hair follicles through which oil flows onto the surface of the skin.

In acne, the oil does not flow freely onto the surface but backs up in the follicles. While we don't know exactly why and how this occurs, we do know that once this happens bacteria in the follicles play a role. These bacteria contain enzymes that break down sebum into free fatty acids that irritate and weaken the walls of the follicles. It is also believed that the lining of hair follicle walls in acne patients is abnormal, so dead cells may accumulate in layers and block up the follicles or pores. This contributes to the formation of blackheads and whiteheads.

As oil continues to flow into the hair follicles and is broken down by bacteria, there is continued irritation that causes the walls to rupture, releasing bacteria and sebum into surrounding tissues and producing inflammation and acne pimples, the next stage of acne. Next pustules and cysts may form.

Broad-spectrum antibiotics such as tetracycline and erythromycin, taken orally, are believed to inhibit bacterial growth within the follicle and to prevent the formation of free fatty acids. Low-dose antibiotic therapy is used by many physicians today to treat selected cases of acne. Antibiotic therapy is recommended for treating severe, inflammatory, recalcitrant acne that does not respond to other measures. It is not usually recommended for mild cases of acne or for pregnant women. Antibiotic therapy has an excellent benefit-to-risk ratio. Among the rare undesirable effects are vaginal moniliasis (yeast infection) among female patients, diarrhea, weight loss, and allergic reactions, including photosensitivity. These problems almost always disappear after antibiotic therapy is stopped. Antibiotics can be continued for months or years, as long as the patient is under the regular, close supervision of a physician.

Except for recent promising trials of lipid soluble antibiotics, such as erythromycin, no evidence exists that topical antibiotic preparations will prevent, relieve, or cure acne.

CRYOSURGERY FOR ACNE

I've heard about a new treatment for acne called cryosurgery. How does it work?

The term cryosurgery refers to a medical treatment that consists of freezing the skin. This treatment is used by physicians to remove certain skin growths, to treat certain skin disorders —including acne—and to improve the appearance of scarring that may result from conditions such as acne. The agents most commonly used for cryosurgery are liquid nitrogen and solid carbon dioxide (dry ice). Carbon dioxide slush (solid carbon ground up and mixed with acetone) is also used. Sulfur is sometimes added to the slush when treating acne. Sprays containing highly volatile solvents are also used to some extent for cryosurgery. The choice of agent depends in part on its availability. For instance, a physician can usually obtain dry ice from several sources, while liquid nitrogen may not be readily available in some locations.

Cryosurgery is by no means a "new" procedure; it has been utilized in various forms for more than thirty years. But not all physicians use the procedure, and some are more enthusiastic than others about its benefits. The choice of cryosurgery over other procedures, and the choice of agent to be used for cryosurgery, is a decision to be made by the physician based on an evaluation of each individual case.

Cryosurgery produces irritation and peeling of the skin, which is considered beneficial for many cases of acne. It also sometimes helps to reduce inflammation (redness) after irritation has subsided. Cryosurgery may reduce the severity of acne scarring, but cannot completely remove acne scars. It may be of help for selected patients when performed by a physician experienced in its use.

ACNE AND VITAMIN E

One friend told me that rubbing vitamin E on my skin would help my acne and the scarring that has resulted from it. Another said I must take vitamin E capsules to obtain any benefit. Who's right?

Neither of your friends is correct. Acne is not caused by any vitamin deficiency, and there is no scientific evidence to support claims that vitamin E is helpful for acne or for acne scarring. In fact, there is no evidence that vitamin E is helpful for any common skin problem.

The fact that a substance is relatively safe when ingested doesn't mean it can be safely applied to the skin. Some people have developed discomforting skin rashes after applying vitamin E oil from capsules. Problems with cosmetic preparations made with vitamin E have also occurred. In one case, the manufacturer of a vitamin E deodorant had to withdraw the product from the market because of consumer complaints about adverse skin reactions.

If you have acne that does not respond to routine skin care, such as frequent cleansing and use of nonprescription products, consult a dermatologist for treatment. There is no cure for acne, but proper treatment can help minimize the severity of the condition and subsequent scarring.

COSMETIC SKIN-PEELING TREATMENTS

What is your opinion of the safety and effectiveness of treatments offered by "beauty treatment" salons for the improvement of acne and acne scarring that involve using 10 percent resorcinol to peel the skin?

Resorcinol is a keratolytic (peeling) agent. In low concentrations (usually 2 percent to 10 percent) it dries and mildly peels the outer layer of the skin, which is considered helpful in treating acne. Thus resorcinol, in low concentrations, is incorporated into many acne treatment preparations prescribed by physicians or sold directly to the public.

In concentrations of 10 percent or more, resorcinol may produce severe irritation, redness, swelling, and deeper peeling. The swelling may temporarily improve the appearance of acne scars and fine lines or wrinkles, but resorcinol at these concentrations may also be harmful.

Scarring, staining, and hyperpigmentation are among the skin problems that may result from improper use of resorcinol.

The chemical may also be absorbed through the skin and thus has the potential to produce internal damage.

A beauty treatment using 10 percent resorcinol is associated with considerable risk and generally is not recommended. Immediately following therapy, the skin will be irritated and look as if it were severely sunburned and peeling. When this wears off, the treated area will be edematous (swollen) and red. If these reactions are severe, they may be cosmetic defects in their own right. The treated areas also may become sun sensitive. Such treatment should be undertaken only by an experienced physician and the patient should be aware of the overall risks involved.

The skin's structure and sensitivity vary widely from one person to another and in different skin areas on the same person, such as the cheeks, neck, and areas around the eyes. Thus the concentration of resorcinol and the length of time it should remain on the skin may vary for different skin areas and for different people. Treatment must be individualized.

TREATMENT FOR ACNE SCARS

Can anything be done to prevent acne scars? What can be done for scars that already exist?

The best way to avoid acne scars is to treat acne properly, and this is best done under a physician's supervision. Severe cases of acne usually require treatment by a specialist. Most important, the prescribed procedures must be carried out faithfully and regularly for the treatments to be successful.

Once acne has subsided, scars already present may be improved, though not totally eliminated, by dermabrasion (skin planing). Dermabrasion is discussed in Chapter 22, "Esthetic Surgery."

14

Aging and Wrinkles

ISOMETRICS FOR AGING SKIN

I read recently that isometric exercises will help improve sagging and wrinkled skin and prevent the appearance of further undesirable changes. Is this true?

No kind of exercise, isometric or otherwise, will erase wrinkles and sagging skin due to aging. Although muscles that move facial skin may be exercised, structural changes associated with aging primarily involve the skin; there is no convincing evidence that increasing the tonicity of such muscles will prevent sagging and flabbiness or improve contour.

Four major changes distinguish the old from the young face. Facial contour changes; natural lines of expression and action of the face and neck deepen and become more obvious; the skin becomes lax and sags into characteristic folds and pouches; and the color of the skin changes.

Medical authorities generally agree that continuous excessive exposure to sunlight also contributes greatly to skin aging. In fact, many physicians believe it may play a greater role than chronological age. Certainly most of the visible signs of aging, including wrinkles, are much more pronounced on areas of the skin exposed to light.

Aging skin in which wrinkles are present shows loss of normal elastic tissue and other degenerative changes. These cannot be reversed by exercises.

WRINKLES AND EXCESSIVE DRYNESS

I am a woman of fifty-five. I wish to prevent my skin from drying up and wrinkling like that of my mother, whom I resemble. What special creams are recommended?

Most changes in the skin that we associate with aging, such as excessive dryness, wrinkling, and spots of hyperpigmentation ("senile freckles"), are limited to exposed areas of the skin and, directly or indirectly, are due to the ultraviolet rays of sunlight.

These changes begin very early in life and, of course, can be exaggerated if a light-skinned person lives in a sunny climate or indulges in excessive sunbathing. Apart from avoiding sun exposure and using sun-protective creams at all times and in all places, beginning in childhood, nothing is known that will reverse such changes.

The only benefits to aging skin that "rejuvenating" creams can provide, regardless of the "exotic" or "active" ingredients they claim to contain, are temporary relief from dryness and temporary softening and smoothing of fine lines and rough skin (see Chapter 2, "Rejuvenating Cosmetics").

Chemical peeling or dermabrasion may partially correct age and ultraviolet induced skin changes, if recommended and performed by a physician experienced in these techniques. Various methods of esthetic surgery are discussed in Chapter 22, "Esthetic Surgery."

MASSAGE OF LITTLE VALUE

Is facial massage of any value? I have heard that it stimulates circulation, thus "toning" and firming the skin to help preserve youthful contours.

There is little or no scientific data to show that facial massage helps prevent the changes that go with aging. Vigorous massage may temporarily increase blood flow to the skin, and even produce some swelling by increasing the amount of fluid in the tissues. However, such a change is certainly not of lasting benefit.

Several so-called facial exercisers or massagers have been developed. The information available on these devices does not support their manufacturers' claims. Several brands have been seized by the Federal Government for false and misleading claims.

VALUE OF FACE MASQUES FOR AGING SKIN

How beneficial are face masques?

Face packs or masques usually contain clays, gums, or synthetic rubber polymers. Clays are the safest and the most popular; rubber polymers present the possibility of causing skin irritation. Some people, particularly those with excessively dry skin, may find the masques irritating; otherwise they are not considered harmful.

Face masques will not rejuvenate aging skin. Many of their benefits are psychological, since the warmth and sense of tightening that occur as the masque dries give a feeling that "something must be happening." When the masque is removed the skin feels refreshed, and there is a cleansing effect in that surface skin debris is removed along with the masque. While these preparations will not provide the degree of benefit implied in advertising, many people are apparently satisfied with the results.

FACIAL SAUNAS FOR AGING SKIN

What is your opinion of the so-called facial sauna devices that claim to benefit aging skin?

These devices were in use in Europe, particularly in Germany and Austria, more than thirty years ago, and have more recently become quite popular in France and the United States. Essentially, they expose the skin to a warm, wet atmosphere—

an effect that can be achieved very easily by applying a warm, wet towel to the face for 5 minutes. This is a method used in barbershops before shaving, and it is certainly most relaxing.

No doubt the device temporarily increases circulation to the skin. It also introduces quite a bit of moisture into the upper layers of the skin surface. But unless this is followed immediately by the application of creams or ointments, the moisture will evaporate within half an hour or so. It would appear that a "facial sauna" is an alternative to applying a hot, wet towel to your face. It has no particular benefit for aging skin and may even further dry the skin.

COD LIVER OIL FOR WRINKLES

I read in a book that cod liver oil will plump out wrinkles. Is this true? How should I use it?

Whether taken internally or applied to the skin, cod liver oil does not "plump out" or remove wrinkles. The application of cod liver oil, mineral oil, baby oil, or any other oil, cream, or lotion will help retard evaporation of moisture, thus temporarily relieving dry skin and making it feel smoother and softer.

Esthetic surgery, either plastic or dermatologic surgery, is the only means of significantly improving wrinkled skin.

TEMPORARY FACELIFTS

A local department store has been selling a variety of head-band devices that are supposed to provide a temporary facelift. Are these effective? Can they be harmful?

The elastic bands or cords you describe are designed to pull up and tighten the skin on the lower part of the face, primarily around the chin, and to produce a general lifting effect. The bands are tied around the head and attached at the temples with adhesive tape or glue; some are also anchored to a section of hair at the back of the head. The bands are supposed to be worn during the day, concealed by hair (or a wig preferably) and makeup.

How effective are these devices? That depends on how well they fit, how adept a person is at applying them and how much "facelifting" the person needs. Many people require a surgical facelift before any significant improvement is apparent.

The bands work primarily on the chin line, and have reportedly been used for some time by television and motion picture personalities. While they are not harmful in themselves, the cords can contribute to headaches if worn too tightly. If you decide to try for your own temporary facelift, ask the store clerk to have someone show you how to properly apply the bands.

WRINKLE TREATMENT WITH ELECTRIC NEEDLE

Do you have any information on the safety and effectiveness of a method of removing wrinkles that involves introducing an electric needle into the skin?

In this technique a needle transmitting an electric current is introduced at an angle just underneath the skin. The current produces considerable swelling (edema), followed by superficial scaling and skin irritation. The swelling tends to smooth out wrinkles. However, after a short time this temporary traumatic effect subsides, and the improvement disappears. If the electric current is too strong it may produce skin irritation, scarring, and hyperpigmentation (dark spots). If you are concerned about wrinkles, we suggest that you consult a physician experienced in esthetic surgery for information about accepted medical procedures that would be beneficial.

SENILE FRECKLES—AGE SPOTS

As I grow older, I have noticed the appearance of brown spots on the backs of my hands and on my face. What causes these spots, and can anything be done to make them go away? Are they dangerous?

Frecklelike brown spots commonly appear on exposed areas of skin such as the backs of the hands, the face, and the neck as a person ages. Although they resemble the freckles of youth, their size and shape are larger and more irregular. Their color is darker and uneven, and they do not fade in winter. These spots are referred to as old-age (senile) freckles, liver spots, or senile lentigines (singular: lentigo).

Regardless of their name, there is no connection between these spots and liver disease, nor is age itself the principal cause. They are caused primarily by years of exposure to sun and wind, and the skin in these areas usually shows other evidence of sun damage.

By the time the brown spots appear, the skin has been irreversibly damaged. Treatment consists of preventing further irritation. Sunbathing and extreme exposure to sunlight should be avoided, and a sun-protective cream should be used when exposure is unavoidable. No perfect bleach cream exists, but various preparations may lighten the color, as discussed in Chapter 1, "Cosmetic Creams."

Self-diagnosis and treatment of pigmented spots is not recommended. Lesions of this type should be examined by a physician if they are enlarging, becoming thicker, or developing a crust, since they may indicate the presence of skin cancer, which may also develop on exposed skin. Physicians have several techniques available for removing such spots.

15

Birthmarks —
Pigmentation Disorders

STRAWBERRY BIRTHMARKS

Our baby has a strawberry birthmark on her face. We would appreciate information on this.

The vascular birthmark (hemangioma) commonly called a strawberry mark may be present at birth or may appear during the first few months of life. It is elevated above the skin's surface, usually has a distinct border and is soft and compressible. A strawberry mark can occur anywhere on the body. Most commonly the lesions are no more than 1 or 2 inches in diameter; however, they can involve an entire extremity.

Usually the lesion grows rapidly for the first several months, during which time it may increase several times in size. After a variable period, during which the size remains unchanged, the lesion begins to fade. As a rule, regression is very slow; 2, 4, or even 6 years may elapse before it disappears completely—but this usually occurs by the time the child is ready for school.

Reliable statistics show complete, spontaneous disappearance of strawberry hemangiomas in 50 percent of patients by age five and 70 percent by age seven; in these patients little if any cosmetic defect remains. Of the hemangiomas that do not regress, less than 10 percent are so cosmetically disturbing that they require treatment. For this reason, many authorities recommend waiting at least 4 years before considering treatment, although some physicians still believe that the birth-mark should be treated immediately to prevent further en-largement.

If you and your physician decide to treat the birthmark, several methods are available. However, all therapy involves some risk, and the cosmetic results may not be as good as those produced by spontaneous regression. Choice of treatment should be left to the judgment of your physician.

PORT-WINE STAINS

Can the birthmark called port-wine stain be treated to lighten or improve its appearance?

Port-wine stain, a form of birthmark (hemangioma) that ap-pears as a flat, bluish-red patch of variable size, is produced by a congenital overgrowth of small blood vessels in the skin.

In contrast to strawberry hemangiomas, port-wine heman-giomas do not clear up spontaneously. Treatment of these birthmarks generally is unsatisfactory because they usually are too large to be removed surgically and do not respond to X-ray or radium treatment.

Some forms of treatment for port-wine stains are super-ficially destructive to the skin, such as freezing with dry ice or dermabrasion (scraping the skin). The patient must realize that such procedures may create cosmetic defects that are rarely less noticeable than the birthmark itself.

Usually, the most successful way to manage a port-wine stain is to use a specially designed masking cream to obscure the lesion. With instructions and practice, a good cosmetic result can be obtained.

TATTOOING FOR PORT-WINE STAINS

How effective is tattooing as a treatment for port-wine stain birthmarks?

Tattooing with skin-colored pigment has sometimes been helpful in treating port-wine stains. However, as stated in the previous answer, there is no way to remove this kind of birthmark completely without leaving other undesirable marks in its place.

Tattooing for port-wine stains is a highly specialized procedure and should always be done by an experienced physician. It is difficult to match natural skin color with tattoo pigments, and the tattooed skin may not match the adjacent skin in all seasons, since tattooed areas do not tan. Thus, both patient and family should be fully aware of the limitations of tattooing.

TREATMENT OF FRECKLES

During the summer my freckles become much more noticeable. How can I tone them down?

Our best advice is to leave them alone. If you avoid sunlight, your freckles will naturally become less evident in time. Much of the success attributed to freckle creams may be due to this natural loss of color. There is little to indicate that the use of any freckle cream for a brief period of time (several weeks) is harmful, unless irritation or allergic reactions occur. However, such creams should not be used for longer periods of time. (Bleaching creams are discussed in more detail in Chapter 1, "Cosmetic Creams.")

THE MASK OF PREGNANCY

I have developed brownish spots and patches on my face since I became pregnant. Will these spots disappear after my baby is born?

Skin discoloration such as you describe is fairly common during pregnancy and is sometimes called "the mask of pregnancy." It results from an increase of pigment, and is most common in brunettes and others with a considerable amount of pigment in their skin.

The discoloration should gradually fade after your baby is born. In the meantime, if the darkened areas bother you, they can be concealed with a masking cosmetic.

This type of skin discoloration may also occur in a small percentage of women who are taking birth control pills, as discussed in the following question and answer.

Pigmentation caused by either pregnancy or oral contraceptives will be intensified by exposure to the sun. To minimize further darkening of pigment, wear a sun block or barrier preparation when you must be out in the sun. A regular suntan preparation will not be effective for this purpose. Your dermatologist can prescribe one that blocks out most of the burning and tanning rays of the sun that darken skin. (Sample brands are also listed in the brand-name guide at the end of Chapter 20, "Sunlight and the Skin.")

BIRTH CONTROL BLOTCHES

I've developed dark blotches on my face from taking birth control pills. How can I get rid of the discoloration? Removal of the skin blotches caused by birth control pills cannot be guaranteed. If you stop taking the pills, the discoloration may fade in 2 or 3 years, but some discoloration may remain. You can try using special bleaching creams that contain hydroquinone or its derivatives. But often it takes many months before any results are noticed, and the creams may cause irritation or allergic reactions. Chemical peeling, which should be performed only by a physician, is not always recommended either. Sometimes it works, but it may have the opposite effect and increase the pigmentation.

Your best bet is camouflage. Ordinary face powders and foundations, however, are not sufficient. Instead, use masking cosmetics under your regular makeup. Because the discoloration is caused by excessive pigmentation, it's also important to protect your skin from the summer sun. Use sunblocking or barrier preparations, instead of suntan lotions, whenever you're outdoors. Avoid sunbathing and wear a hat with a wide brim. Direct sunlight will only intensify the blotches.

The discoloration you describe is the same as "the mask of pregnancy" that often affects pregnant women. Thus "The Pill," which creates a condition comparable to pregnancy, can cause the same blotches, known as chloasma or melasma. For the most part, dark-complexioned women are more susceptible than those with fair skin.

CAUSE OF WHITE SKIN PATCHES

I have developed white patches of skin on my arms and legs that are most distressing since I am black. What causes these patches?

You would have to consult a physician to discover the cause of your particular problem. Several disorders cause a lessening of skin pigment that can be interpreted as a loss of pigment. Normal skin color is produced by a pigment called melanin. When the skin stops producing melanin—often for unknown reasons—smooth, light-colored patches develop. Depigmentation of this type can be produced by chemicals contained in some rubber products and certain brands of tape, as well as by other agents and skin disorders.

These white patches are not harmful or contagious but can be a significant cosmetic defect, especially when the skin is dark. Unfortunately, no completely satisfactory medical or cosmetic treatment has been found, as discussed in the following question and answer.

TREATMENT OF WHITE SKIN PATCHES

Can white skin patches be removed from dark-skinned persons?

Unfortunately, there is no completely satisfactory medical or cosmetic treatment available today for lightened skin patches.

Most often, medical treatments are directed at stimulating repigmentation with drugs called psoralens. These drugs are administered orally, after which the skin is exposed to a prescribed amount of sunlight or blacklight fluorescent light. The process is long, tedious, and time consuming, with no guarantee of complete effectiveness, but varying amounts of repigmentation can occur. In some cases, this treatment has enabled patients to return to normal roles in society, although not all affected areas become equally repigmented.

In a few cases where most of the skin has become depigmented, physicians have removed the pigment from the few remaining spots of normal skin so that all of the skin is a lighter color. But this treatment is controversial and the results are not always predictable.

Articles in the lay press have reported that the drug used in this process can be used generally to lighten dark-colored skin. This, however, is not the case. The treatment is suitable only for patients who are seriously affected by light blotches and have only a few areas of normally pigmented skin remaining. Even then it is not considered a routine procedure.

The most practical approach may be to simply camouflage the patches. Try either natural or synthetic stains, available from your physician or pharmacist. The lightened patches can also be covered or "masked" with special heavy cosmetics designed for covering birthmarks. They come in various makeup shades and are available at many cosmetic counters.

TREATMENT OF VITILIGO

Please discuss recent advances concerning a cure or help for vitiligo patients. Are preparations available to improve the appearance of skin in the areas involved? Is the cause of this skin disease known?

Vitiligo is a condition of unknown cause in which certain areas of the skin fail to produce melanin, the pigment responsible for normal skin color. Light-colored patches of skin form as a result. While vitiligo is seen in all races, it is naturally a greater cosmetic defect when the skin is dark.

In recent years, considerable interest has been shown in using drugs called psoralens to treat this condition. Repigmentation can occur in varying degrees when they are taken orally and their ingestion is followed by daily exposure to sunlight or ultraviolet light. However, the treatment must be continued over a long period, is very tedious and time consuming, and in many patients results have been only fair and transient. Many patients and many skin areas do not respond. Any patient taking psoralens must be under medical supervision.

Another useful approach in treating vitiligo is to camouflage the lesions, thus improving cosmetic appearance. Suitable preparations include various natural and synthetic stains available through physicians and pharmacies, and special nonprescription cosmetics designed to cover birthmarks.

CHANGING SKIN COLOR

Can dark-skinned people lighten their skin significantly by using bleaching creams or by any other method?

Basic skin color is genetically determined, and the amount of normal pigment skin contains cannot be permanently altered. Bleaching creams of all kinds are worthless for this purpose.

16

Dry Skin,
Oily Skin

DRY SKIN

What causes dry skin?
Many factors influence the dryness of skin: age, geographical location, time of year, relative humidity in living and working quarters, and excessive use of soaps and detergents. Individual variations under similar circumstances probably indicate hereditary differences. Dryness of the skin is primarily due to loss of water from the skin's horny outer layer and insufficient movement of moisture upward from lower tissue layers.

In experiments with thin sections of dry and brittle horny tissue, contact with various "fatty" materials such as lanolin or vegetable oil did not restore the pliability of the material even when contact was prolonged. On the other hand, immersing the tissue in water or maintaining it in humid air did. This is the main reason modern cosmetic formulas are designed to provide "moisturizing" action.

AIR CONDITIONING AND DRY SKIN

I work and live in an air-conditioned environment. Can this contribute to dry skin and the formation of premature wrinkles?
To answer this question, it is necessary to define air conditioning. The late Dr. Willis Carrier, who first laid down the en-

gineering principles of air conditioning in 1911, gave this definition: "Air conditioning is the control of the humidity of air by either increasing or decreasing its moisture content. Added to the control of humidity is the control of temperature by either heating or cooling the air, the purification of the air by washing or filtering, and the control of air motion and ventilation."

Air conditioning in large offices and public buildings usually performs all of these functions on a year-round basis. However, air conditioning in many homes and apartment buildings is limited to cooling, purifying, and reducing humidity; heating and adding moisture are not included, and the environment may be air conditioned only during certain periods such as the summer. Few persons live in a constantly air-conditioned environment.

A drop in humidity dries the skin because its moisture escapes into the drier atmosphere. It has been shown that constant exposure to air conditioning produces excessively dry skin in a few individuals, particularly if they are near the draft of air outlets. Excessively dry skin may lead to fine superficial lines; however, this is not an important factor in the formation of premature wrinkles.

People who tend to develop excessively dry skin from air conditioning usually have a preexisting history of dermatitis (skin inflammation). These persons may also tend to wash too frequently, which could add to their skin problems. Air conditioning is definitely beneficial for certain skin conditions such as miliaria (prickly heat), which is discussed in detail in Chapter 21, "Other Skin Problems."

DRY SKIN IN WINTER

I live in a northern city, and in the winter my skin becomes so dry and flaky it feels like sandpaper. Is there anything I can do to prevent this?

In cold climates, dry, flaky, itchy skin during the winter

months may have several causes. Cold, dry outdoor weather and dry, overheated indoor air are the major culprits. Cold wind, excessive use of soaps and detergents, and too frequent bathing in very hot water also take a toll. Of course, aging and heredity have an effect on the skin that is not helped by unfriendly weather.

Almost everyone—particularly older people—could have softer, smoother skin if they didn't bathe so frequently in winter. Take fewer, faster baths; don't use hot, hot water and you won't wash all the moisture out of the outer layer of your skin.

If your skin feels dry, use moisturizing creams or lotions on it every day. These emollient preparations make skin soft and pliable by retarding evaporation of moisture.

Apply body lotions after every bath and each night before you go to bed. Don't forget to put some on your arms and legs—they need special attention. Bath oils are useful too, and will help keep your skin from itching.

By all means women should remember to apply a foundation cream under makeup to protect skin from the cold wind. If your skin is very dry, use only a cream makeup. Skip the powder, and try alternating the use of cleansing cream with soap and water, because soap may have a drying effect on your skin.

DRY SKIN AND FREQUENT BATHS

I've always thought a person should take a bath or shower at least once a day to be clean, but a friend told me that daily baths are unnecessary, especially during the winter for people of my age (seventy-two). My friend says too much bathing may be the cause of my dry, itchy skin. Is this true?

Your friend is probably correct. Too frequent bathing is one of the common causes of dry, itchy skin during the winter, especially in older persons (see previous answer).

Daily sponge baths with tub baths or showers once or twice a week are usually adequate to keep skin clean and odor free. One alternative is a quick daily shower, limiting the use of soap to underarm, genital, and foot areas. It is also advisable to take shorter baths and showers with warm rather than hot water when your skin is excessively dry and itchy.

Daily use of emollient creams and lotions is recommended; bath oils are also helpful supplements when bathing. Be sure to apply a lubricating lotion after bathing and before bedtime. Legs and arms usually need special attention. Frequent, liberal lubrication of your skin may enable you to enjoy the luxury of bathing more often.

Remember that itching can be one symptom of some internal diseases. If itching is general and persistent, consult your physician.

HOW TO RAISE HUMIDITY

Does it help raise humidity in a house and prevent dry skin to place open containers of water near radiators?

Low humidity does contribute to dry skin, but moisture released into the air from evaporation usually is not sufficient to have a significant effect on the relative humidity of a room during the dry winter months. However, if the containers of water have a fairly large surface and are placed against or on top of heating devices (radiators, etc.) evaporation may increase humidity to some extent.

A steam-generating device or humidifier will do a better job of raising relative humidity. Two types of humidifiers are available—hot steam, which produces a small stream of water vapor, and "cold steam," which produces a cloud of very fine water droplets with a small, high-speed turbine. A small, 1-gallon capacity hot steam vaporizer will adequately humidify an average size room for 8 to 10 hours. "Cold-steam" humidifiers are more expensive and unavoidably produce a humming noise because of the high-speed motor.

CARE OF OILY SKIN

Please advise me regarding skin care and cosmetics for oily skin.

Oily skin is a subjective situation: different people "tolerate" varying degrees of oiliness, and oiliness varies in the same person with changes in sun, wind, temperature and emotions. Much depends on the amount of moisture on the skin. The skin's surface oil will spread out on a film of water in much the same way that a drop of motor oil spreads on the surface of a pond. Therefore, in summer when sweating is active, the skin will appear to be more oily.

External applications cannot control the amount of oil that is constantly being delivered to the skin surface, but much of the accumulated material can be removed with soap and water. Most cases are controlled adequately with cleansing three or four times daily.

When washing is inconvenient, as it is at school or at work, an astringent preparation or premoistened packaged cleansing pads can be used. Complexion brushes or abrasive soaps, if used frequently, may irritate the skin, and they offer no advantage for removing surface oil.

Advertising claims, old wives' tales, and misinformation have led many people to think that external oiliness will prevent aging and wrinkles. This is not true, and it should not deter anyone from cleansing adequately for good health and comfort.

Women often want to know what type of cosmetics they should use for oily skin. Obviously, oils and oil-like substances are not recommended; these preparations may only add to the problem. Loose powder and nonoily foundation lotions will meet the needs of most women with oily skin. However, the final judgment of any cosmetic is dictated by the comfort, "feel," and satisfaction it provides.

"COMBINATION" COMPLEXIONS

My complexion is dry in some areas and oily in others. What type of skin care is recommended?
Many women complain that they have both dry and oily skin, causing some difficulty in their selection of proper cosmetic preparations.

In this condition, referred to as "combination" skin, there is a much greater concentration of active oil glands in the mid-forehead, nose, and chin than in the cheeks and temples. Thus the face may have an oily area between excessively dry sides. The use of lubricating (oily) cosmetics may make the center too oily, while "drying" or "defatting" agents may irritate the sides of the face.

In addition, oiliness and dryness vary at different times of the year. Skin tends to be much drier during cold weather, when the humidity is lower. Normal skin may become irritated or rough in winter, then oily in the summer heat when humidity is higher.

What some people consider dry skin may in fact be scales that result from inflammation associated with excessive oiliness—for example, dandruff flaking and seborrheic dermatitis of oily facial areas.

Proper care of "combination" skin requires flexible use of facial cosmetics. Washing with a moderately drying soap two or three times a day and use of a nongreasy cleanser will decrease oiliness in the center areas of your face. Excessive dryness on the sides of your cheeks, your temples and eyelids may be relieved by a lubricating cream, applied sparingly once or twice daily. If excessive oiliness persists, an astringent solvent may be used two or three times daily on your forehead, nose, and chin.

No single cosmetic will care for all skin areas of people

with combination skin. If your problem is serious or disturbing, you should consult a dermatologist, who may be able to increase the effectiveness of your cosmetics by adding more active agents.

OILY NOSE

My nose becomes shiny and oily even though the rest of my face is dry. How can I correct this condition?

This is a fairly common form of "combination complexion," especially in summer (see previous answer). Avoid using oily cleansers and night creams in the nose area. If excessive oiliness persists, an astringent preparation may be used two or three times a day. Don't try to cover up an oily nose by heavy use of cosmetics.

SEBORRHEIC DERMATITIS ON FACE

I have seborrheic dermatitis on my face. I would appreciate any information available about this condition.

Seborrhea refers to a condition in which the sebaceous (oil) glands of the skin produce an excessive amount of sebum (oil). Seborrhea most often occurs on the scalp and face, as the oil glands in these areas are especially plentiful and active. Seborrhea may consist simply of an excessively oily complexion and hair; more severe forms may cause scaling, irritation, and inflammation of the skin and scalp and are referred to as seborrheic dermatitis. The latter usually requires a physician's attention for proper treatment.

Washing your face two or three times a day with moderately drying soap will help control excessive oiliness. Drying and peeling preparations also help. Frequent shampooing is recommended.

Defatting agents such as rubbing alcohol can be used to remove excess oil from your face between washings; premoistened, packaged cleansing pads are useful and convenient to carry. Loose powder and nonoily, light liquid makeup are preferable to cream or heavy cake makeup; obviously, oils and creams should be avoided.

TREATING ENLARGED PORES

I am in my early thirties. The pores on my cheeks have enlarged so much that my skin looks pitted. What causes this condition, and what can I do to improve it?

An enlarged pore is the opening of a hair follicle that usually has a tiny invisible hair and a large, active sebaceous (oil) gland. Enlarged pores are most obvious on the nose and the inner aspect of the cheeks and chin where oil glands are concentrated. Oily skin and, during adolescence, acne usually accompany enlarged pores, and these conditions often recur after middle age.

Nothing can change the size of enlarged pores or prevent more, so don't believe claims that any product or treatment will "shrink" them.

However, cosmetic preparations can help improve your appearance temporarily. Astringent preparations, which usually contain alcohol as the chief ingredient, help remove excess oil and may make the pores less obvious for a short time. Face masks or facials do the same thing. Carefully selected and applied makeup can help conceal enlarged pores. You may have to try several different makeup bases to find the one best suited for you. Generally, for oily skin a liquid base is preferred to a cream base.

CLOSING THE PORES

I have often heard people say that a hot shower followed by a cold one will close the pores of your skin. Is this true? Is it beneficial?

There is no scientific basis for this statement. Pores are the opening onto the skin's surface of sweat glands, oil glands and hair follicles; their size cannot be altered, nor can they be opened and closed.

The "enlarged pore" that is often of cosmetic concern is the opening of a hair follicle that has a very fine, almost invisible hair and a large oil gland.

Astringents may make enlarged pores temporarily less obvious by irritating the surrounding skin so that it swells slightly around the pore.

When you take a hot bath or shower, the heat may increase circulation slightly by causing small blood vessels close to the skin surface to dilate. A cold shower immediately afterward will constrict the blood vessels and may feel good— but it serves no other purpose.

Inflammation such as occurs with sunburn may cause swelling (edema) of the skin, making pores appear smaller for a short period only.

17

Hand, Nail,
and Foot Problems

SPLITTING AND GROOVING OF NAILS

During the past year a decided, gradual grooving has been occurring across my fingernails, which causes splitting and peeling of the nails' ends. Is this serious?

The fingernail is formed by special cells found in the lunula (the white half-moon-shaped portion of the nail). This extends underneath the skin at the base of the nail. Any change in the cells that form the nail may be reflected by changes in the nail's appearance. For instance, inflammation in the region of the skin at the base of the nail may be reflected by a deformity of the nail.

A previous injury, even minor, may also lead to transverse grooving and/or splitting. Thus, while ridging may occur naturally, it is important to determine whether a previous injury to the nail has occurred or inflammation is present that could account for the condition. Since the nail originates far back under the skin (almost to the region of the last finger joint), inflammation of this area, such as arthritis, may also cause mild deformities.

Treatment of any inflammation or other underlying cause may result in improvement in the nail structure. However, because the fingernail takes approximately 3 to 6 months to grow, any improvement in underlying conditions will require that length of time to appear.

The best way to prevent splitting and peeling is to cut your nails short so that they are not pulled away and do not catch against objects.

WHITE SPOTS ON NAILS

What causes white spots on the nails? Are they serious? The nails and hair consist of keratin, a "dead," tough protein substance. The keratinized visible portion of the nail is called the nail plate.

The structure of the nail plate itself and its attachments to underlying tissues determine the color of the nail. The nail takes its origin from the semilunar white region at the base of the nail plate called the lunula. The lunula is present in all nails, although it may be hidden under the skin at the base of the nail in the fourth and fifth digits. Cells in the lunula are still undergoing keratinization and reflect white light. As the nail grows out, these cells become fully hardened and the whiteness disappears.

Whenever keratinization of the cells forming the nail plate is incomplete or changed, white spots or streaks result. These spots are rather common and have developed a rich folklore, under such names as gift spots, lies, sweethearts, and fortune spots.

Usually, the white spots result from minor trauma in the body of the nail such as may occur during manicuring. However, they can result from any disturbance to the lunula. In some instances, the white spots arise from a fungus infection and require the attention of a physician. Otherwise, small spots probably require no treatment.

The nail may also appear white if it is separated from its nail bed. That is why the end of the nail is white. Any disorder, therefore, that causes separation of the nail creates a white area, which may be a signal for medical attention.

BRITTLE NAILS

What can be done for brittle, splitting fingernails?
The exact cause of most cases of brittle nails is not known. They probably are due not to internal factors, but to external agents such as detergents, cleansers, and solvents contained in polish removers. Nail brittleness also increases with age.

We are not aware of any effective therapy for brittle nails. Although many commercial products are marketed for this purpose, their effectiveness has not been proved. Some studies appear to indicate improvement following daily ingestion of large doses of gelatin, but evidence is not sufficient to support the value of this remedy.

A few years ago, nail hardeners with formaldehyde as the active ingredient were introduced. These are discussed in detail in Chapter 4, "Reactions to Cosmetics."

Creams and oils for nails are also available. These preparations applied to nails every few days will help counteract surface drying but will not cure brittle nails.

A woman can do several things to prevent or minimize nail damage: wear rubber gloves with cotton linings whenever possible while performing "wet" household work; and use a hand cream regularly, massaging it into the skin around the nails. Nail polish or nail-coating products can act as a splint or shield to protect nails. Some nail polishes contain nylon fibers that thicken and thereby strengthen nails. Nail polish should not be removed too frequently because of the drying effect of polish remover. It's better to patch chips that may occur.

If brittleness occurs without known external cause, or is persistent and severe, see your doctor.

PREVENTING HANGNAILS

I have a lot of trouble with hangnails. What can I do to correct or prevent them?

Hangnails are splits in the skin along the sides of the nails, often resulting from excessive dryness of the skin in these areas. Dried skin loses its elasticity and tends to crack. Hangnails may also develop from picking the skin around the nail, from inexpert manicuring, or from accidental injury such as cuts from the edge of a piece of paper. These small fissured areas are annoying and often painful.

The main cause of excessive dryness is repeated washing and inadequate drying of hands. To prevent hangnails, wear cotton-lined rubber gloves when washing dishes or clothes, and always dry hands thoroughly. Careful manicuring and the use of emollient creams or ointments several times a day also help prevent hangnails. If a hangnail develops, the tip of dry skin should be cut off carefully, rather than pulled, thus avoiding injury to live skin.

FUNGAL INFECTIONS OF THE NAILS

I have a fungal infection of my toenails. What treatment is recommended?

Fungal infections of the nails may be caused by several fungi including the common tinea fungus responsible for athlete's foot or by a yeastlike fungus. The nails become thickened, moist, discolored, and sometimes have pus underneath. Inflammation of the skin surrounding the nail may take place, with pus formation. The nail may also be separated from its base. Toenails may become so greatly enlarged and distorted that discomfort and pain result, especially when pressure is placed on the nails by the wearing of shoes.

Nails infected with fungi are a unique problem. The infections respond very poorly, if at all, to mere surface application of remedies. Persistent scraping and clipping to remove as much of the infected nail as possible is essential to the treatment routine. In this process, much of the nail plate and the accumulated scale under it may be removed. Surgical removal of the nail fails to bring about cure in most cases.

Many people may not wish to invest the time and effort required to cure fungal infections of the nails, but a regimen of persistent trimming and scraping will at least prevent thickening, distortion, and discomfort. For a few selected individuals with significant symptoms due to extensive nail infection caused by certain fungi, long-term treatment with oral medication in conjunction with appropriate local treatment is sometimes undertaken.

DISCOLORATION OF NAILS

What causes persistent dark discoloration of the nails?
This may result from various skin or internal disorders, from infection, or from contact with a variety of compounds and chemicals.

If the nail plate is deeply stained, discoloration will remain until a new nail has grown. Nail hardeners, hair dyes, topical medications, nail polish, cigarette smoking, and numerous other things have been blamed for this sort of discoloration. Nails may also acquire a blue-black or grayish discoloration following any prolonged stress that interferes with nail formation.

You may have to consult a physician for an accurate diagnosis of your condition. Once the underlying cause is determined and removed, nails will begin to grow normally. Nails grow very slowly, however, so it may take 6 months for complete replacement of discolored nails.

In the meantime, if nail polish is not the cause of the discoloration, it may be used as a camouflage.

NAIL CARE FOR YOUNG MEN

My eighteen-year-old son persistently has trouble with his cuticles because he picks his fingernails and doesn't take care of his hands properly. How can I teach him proper care of his hands and nails?
Teaching young men proper care of nails can be difficult because they often consider it unmasculine to use manicuring

equipment and preparations. This idea should be overcome, since attractive, well-groomed nails are as important to men as to women.

Keeping the cuticles pushed back against the base of the nail helps minimize the temptation to pick at them, which makes them ragged and torn. The cuticle can be softened by washing, then gently pushed back against the base of the nail with a manicuring stick or with gentle pressure of the thumbnail of the opposite hand. Overly aggressive manicuring practices may damage the cuticles and nails, so manicuring should be carried out carefully.

Sometimes it is better to avoid doing anything to the cuticle tissue in an effort to divert attention away from the area. If the cuticle is left alone, the tissue will heal and may no longer present a problem.

Your son should learn to use an emery board or fingernail file to smooth the rough edges of his nails so he won't be tempted to bite them. Nails should be filed gently and the edges beveled by passing the fine side of the emery board, held at a 45° angle, around the edge.

Your son's nails should always be filed before he washes his hands, when they are hard and firm, and should be carefully cut with scissors or nail clippers only after a warm bath, when they are soft and pliable.

HOUSEWIVES' DERMATITIS

I am a housewife and find it difficult to avoid skin irritation on my hands. What do you advise?

Skin irritation on hands is so common among housewives that doctors refer to it as "housewives' dermatitis." It is commonly believed that household soaps and detergents, particularly those used for dishwashing and laundering, are the primary cause of this problem. However, in many cases other factors may be involved.

This problem usually occurs during winter months, when

atmospheric temperature and humidity are low. Repeated exposure to water itself makes the skin more susceptible to irritation by common substances that might not ordinarily affect it. Repeated wetting and drying alters the natural defenses of the outermost layers of skin, so that substances commonly encountered in household work such as foods, laundry, soils, household chemicals, and polishes can penetrate the skin more easily and cause irritation. Preexisting skin problems and minor abrasions, as well as bacterial and fungal infections, may also play a role.

Although the setting in which housewives' dermatitis occurs is complex, a woman can do many things to prevent or minimize irritation. The problem usually begins with small, dry, red, and scaly patches, which in early stages are frequently indistinguishable from chapping. Or there may be irritation beneath a ring or around the fingernails.

At this point it often helps to avoid wetting your hands frequently. Wash your hands as seldom as possible, and if washing dishes, laundering, and other tasks involving water cannot be avoided, wear cotton gloves with rubber gloves over them.

Whenever your hands must be wet, rinse them with lukewarm water, dry them thoroughly, and apply an emollient hand cream or lotion. The emollient should be used frequently and applied liberally before bedtime. Cotton gloves or liners can be worn over the cream so that it won't rub off on clothing, bedding, or other objects. In addition, guard against minor injuries such as cuts and burns, which also make skin more susceptible to irritation.

If, despite preventive measures and emollients, your skin problem persists or worsens, consult your physician.

CRACKED SKIN ON FINGERS

What causes cracked skin on the fingers around the nails? I wear gloves outdoors and use creams, but the problem persists.

Cracked skin around the fingers and nails has a number of causes. The most common is exposure to some irritant or allergen. Chapping due to cold and dryness may also contribute to the condition. Occupational exposure, either household or industrial, or an allergy to nail preparations such as cuticle removers, nail polish, or base coats could be the cause. Even the games people play (for instance, contact with an allergen or irritant in picking up playing cards from a wooden, lacquered, or plastic table top) may create this condition.

In other cases external causes are not the source of irritation; diseases or disturbances in circulation bring on the condition.

A cure is usually not possible until you discover and eliminate the cause, and this may require a great deal of detective work. Since gloves and creams have not produced results, the best advice is to see a skin specialist who has the time and interest to investigate the possible causes.

DERMATITIS FROM RINGS

The skin under and around my wedding ring is red and irritated. Does this mean that I'm allergic to the metal in the ring—and will I have to stop wearing it?
Your skin reaction may be a form of "housewives' hands," which often starts under the rings a woman wears. This rarely reflects an allergy to wedding rings. However, reactions under inexpensive rings may be caused by an allergic sensitivity to nickel. (Sterling silver and 14- or 18-karat gold do not contain nickel.)

The skin irritation you describe is probably a reaction to soap, detergent, and other cleansers or potentially irritating materials that become trapped under your rings. Even a mild toilet soap, when caught and retained under a ring, can start a dermatitis. A recess around the stone setting in a ring is particularly likely to trap substances that may collect and become concentrated.

To prevent skin irritation, either remove your rings before performing tasks or remove and clean them afterward.

Waterproof gloves may offer some protection. But although they prevent contact with irritating detergents, cleansers, bleaches, and polishes, these gloves may cause other harm by accumulating sweat. Since a waterproof glove prevents evaporation of sweat, wear thin cotton gloves under the rubber gloves to absorb some of the moisture. Waterproof gloves, even cotton lined, should not be worn for more than 15 to 20 minutes at a time to prevent irritation caused by accumulation of sweat.

DISHWASHING DETERGENTS AND HANDS

Do some dishwashing detergents actually make hands soft and smooth?

It is extremely unlikely that any detergent will make your hands soft or smooth. If anything, the reverse is true. Dishwashing detergents are efficient cleansers for dishes, but they're not good for skin.

Whether or not you get "dishpan hands" probably depends on your own susceptibility—dry skin, allergies, use of too much soap or detergent, or exposure to substances that remove skin oils and dry your skin—rather than on what brand of detergent you use.

The skin of the hands tolerates a great variety of potentially irritating substances. However, everyone's skin has a breaking point and may at some time become irritated. Once your skin is injured, it can't tolerate as much as it could before, and should not come in contact with irritating substances if it is to heal.

Suffice it to say that although detergents, properly used, can be tolerated by most of us, they offer no therapeutic benefits.

RELIEF FOR ACHING FEET

How valuable are foot lotions and/or foot baths for relieving tired, aching feet that result from a day of walking or shopping?

It has been estimated that 70 to 80 percent of women and 60 to 70 percent of men have foot problems. Proper foot care and well-fitted shoes, socks, and stockings are the most important factors in general foot care. Consult a physician about problems such as fungal infections (athlete's foot), ingrown toenails, calluses, corns, deformities, etc., because these require medical attention. Self-medication may only make such conditions worse. (Questions and answers about some of these problems follow.)

The primary cause of tired, sore, aching feet should be determined in order to correct the condition. Keep activities such as shopping or walking to a tolerable level to prevent problems, but when tired, aching feet do occur, rest your feet in an elevated position for temporary relief.

Cosmetic foot preparations are also available for temporary relief; foot lotions similar to regular astringent preparations have a pleasant, cooling and relaxing effect. Deodorizing ingredients are sometimes added to combat foot odors.

Foot powders are similar to regular talcum and body powders except that they may be heavier in texture and more absorbent. Various ingredients are often added for antiseptic and astringent effects; menthol may be included to provide a pleasant fragrance and a cooling, soothing feeling. Foot powders are manufactured mainly to relieve soreness and tenderness by lubricating the feet, preventing chafing, absorbing perspiration, and retarding excess perspiration.

Aerosol foot preparations (lotions or powders in pressurized form) are gaining in popularity. Their advantages are primarily cosmetic: the pressurized package provides a clean and easy method of application.

Foot baths prepared from foot-bath salts may provide excellent relief for tired, aching, sore feet. Hot-water soaks or baths increase the local blood supply and promote circulation, relieving soreness in the feet. The alkali in the salts helps soften the outer horny layers of skin and facilitates the removal of stale secretions, debris, and possible sources of odor.

Other products on the market for relief of minor foot problems include creams, salves, ointments, and balms. A cold cream or a vanishing cream base may be used for foot ointments and with other ingredients can provide a soothing and cooling effect on feet.

PREVENTING FOOT PROBLEMS

How can I prevent foot problems such as bunions, calluses, and corns?

One of the first ways to prevent most foot problems is to wear properly fitting shoes, but it appears that few people do. A dermatologist, reviewing foot problems at a medical meeting, stated that many foot ailments are the result of squeezing youngsters' feet into short shoes. He added that this applies to a large percentage of the total population today.

A survey of 2,000 school children in Denmark disclosed that 79 percent were wearing shoes too small for them. A study in Manchester, England turned up the fact that 48 percent of the young girls studied had "bad feet" by the time they were ten. And, to illustrate how early it all starts, one kindergarten group of fifty-six had only five youngsters wearing properly fitted shoes. Deformities of the great toes, bunions, hammertoes, corns, ingrown toenails, and nail dystrophy are among the headaches—or foot aches—that this can cause.

SOCKS AND FOOT PROBLEMS IN CHILDREN

My eight-year-old daughter has been bothered by athlete's foot for years. Could wearing socks reinforced with nylon toes be the cause? How should this condition be treated?

If by the term "athlete's foot" you mean a fungal infection of the feet, this could not have been caused by socks reinforced with nylon toes. Furthermore, a fungal infection confined to the feet and lasting for many years is rare in an eight-year-old girl. Many more common skin diseases cause scaling, redness, blistering, and soreness of the feet. Diagnosis by a skin specialist should be established before treatment is advised.

Nylon reinforcement in the toes of socks can aggravate fungal infections and other skin diseases of the feet because the fabric is not absorbent. While no evidence exists that a truly allergic reaction is ever caused by nylon itself, the fabric finishes used on nylon and other synthetic fibers have been known to cause dermatitis in rare instances. The diagnosis can be established in individual cases only by specialized procedures.

ROUGH SKIN ON HEELS

Are any creams or cosmetics available today that are effective in removing rough skin from heels?

Preparations advertised to remove rough skin from heels are of two general types: emollient skin lotions or creams, and medicated preparations containing a keratolytic (peeling) agent. The first type is usually harmless and may actually soften dry, chapped skin; the latter type, if improperly used, can frequently cause more trouble than it relieves.

During bathing, when rough skin and calluses are softened by warm water, gentle scrubbing with a soft brush or gentle rubbing with a pumice stone (powdered volcanic glass pressed into textured, solid form) will help remove dead skin and calloused spots. After bathing, massage a mild cream or lotion into the areas.

For mild conditions of roughness, which anyone may experience from time to time, a regular hand lotion, body lotion or cold cream is probably as effective as anything else. For more extreme and persistent conditions, consult a physician.

CALLUSES ON THE FEET

What causes calluses on feet? How can they be removed? Calluses are distinctly thickened areas of skin that usually result from chronic rubbing of shoes over a bony prominence. They are very much like corns, but do not have the regular, round shape of corns or the core. Caused by friction and pressure, calluses are commonly a device of the body to protect the soft, sensitive flesh beneath them. Callus formation may be preceded by a blister. The predisposition to form calluses varies from person to person.

On the feet, calluses typically occur over the area where the plantar fat pad is located. With advancing age, this ordinarily prominent pad atrophies; friction and pressure from walking may then cause a large callus to develop in this area. Calluses may occur on other areas of the foot where bones are prominent, especially over arthritic joints, deviated great toes, and the dorsa of hammertoes. Calluses also develop on areas where the skin becomes folded. Even comparatively young persons can develop calluses on their heels.

When a woman wears high heels her feet are thrust forward, shifting an abnormal amount of weight to the balls of the feet. The constant pressure of this weight can cause painful calluses on the balls of the feet.

No matter what the cause, treatment of a callus should start with elimination of the unnatural friction or pressure that caused it in the first place. This may mean redistributing weight in a more natural pattern. Shoe styles may have to be changed. Padding around the callus will help relieve the pressure on it. The callus itself can usually be removed by soaking and then rubbing it down with pumice. In other cases, keratolytic (peeling) ointments are helpful. Anyone can do this at home, but if cutting is necessary it should be done only by a qualified professional. Therapy should not be too energetic because calluses are actually protective in nature.

INGROWN TOENAILS

What causes ingrown toenails? How can they be treated and prevented?

An ingrown toenail forms when the edge of the nail penetrates adjoining soft tissue. The first symptoms are pain and redness, followed by swelling and discharge. Without proper care, severe infection may follow.

Ill-fitting shoes are the most frequent cause of ingrown toenails. Other factors include poorly trimmed nails (cut too short and too far back at the corner), flat feet, excessive curvature of the nail, obesity, and heredity (having inherited "too large" a big toe, for example). To treat and prevent ingrown nails, wear shoes that are wide enough and long enough not to put pressure on your toes, and don't cut the tips of your toenails. They should be cut across, preferably with clippers, and with the sharp corners only slightly rounded.

To treat a mild case, apply wet dressings and carefully lift and pare off the excess nail. Also, pack sterile cotton under the affected edge of the nail to keep it from penetrating the soft tissue. This should be done daily for at least one week and may cause some discomfort. If the soft tissue surrounding the nail becomes inflamed, soak your foot at least once daily in a hot bath. But if the area becomes infected, see a doctor.

CORNS

I have corns on both of my little toes. I pare them down, but they keep coming back and are painful. What causes corns and what do you suggest for treatment?

A corn is a cone-shaped overgrowth of horny skin with a central hard core. Corns usually occur over bony prominences (such as toe joints) or between the toes, and result from chronic rubbing or pressure for prolonged periods. Improperly fitted shoes are the most common cause, but such growths may also result from disorders such as arthritis, from feet that are off balance, from improperly positioned toes, or from bony spurs that push up against the skin.

Sometimes the point of a corn reaches all the way to the joint below and irritates it until bursitis develops. Bursitis is an inflammation of the bursa, the fluid-filled sac that lubricates the joints. This involvement with the bursa is one of the reasons corns may hurt so much.

You can take positive steps to prevent corns. Since in most cases they are caused by improperly fitted shoes, be sure your shoes do not rub against your toes. Usually the first and fifth toes are the ones affected by corns because shoes may pinch these toes in.

If the corn is caused by a foot that is off balance, this can usually be corrected by professionally trained individuals who understand the mechanics of the feet. Molds that fit into the shoe or pads that lift the foot in certain places and lower it in others (and thus prevent the friction that causes the corn) may be recommended.

Temporary relief from corns can be obtained with flannel pads that fit around them. This takes the pressure off the corn itself.

If you already have corns, seek medical treatment. Self-treatment by paring can lead to more problems because of the underlying bony prominences or, if the person has diabetes, advanced arteriosclerosis or other diseases that affect circulation. Periodic treatments by a qualified physician usually result in alleviation of symptoms. In rare instances, orthopedic surgery on the underlying bones is required.

SOFT CORNS

I have little bumps between my toes that someone told me are corns. What treatment is recommended?

Corns most often occur on the outside of the toe, but they may also occur between the toes. Such whitened and soggy growths occur in the web spaces between toes and are called soft corns. The most common location is between the fourth and fifth toes. These corns are soft because of moisture, and may develop as a result of overriding and frictional pressure between a prominent bump at the joint on one toe and a comparable prominence at the joint of an adjacent toe. Persistence of frictional pressure, often aggravated by the narrowness of highly stylized shoes, may so cramp the fourth and fifth toes that a sinus tract forms and perforates the center of the corn. Some soft corns have been attributed to fungal infections.

Soft corns can be given "first aid" by drying the affected web spaces and by separating the affected toes with padding or lamb's wool. The local use of rubbing alcohol or drying powders plus the wearing of suitable shoes is often helpful. However, professional care is frequently needed to alleviate symptoms caused by the corn or to treat secondary infection, in addition to treating the underlying cause.

CAUSE OF ATHLETE'S FOOT

What causes athlete's foot? Is it true that you usually catch athlete's foot from contact with someone who has it?

The term "athlete's foot" was coined by an advertising man in the 1930s to promote a patent remedy for fungal infections of the feet.

Fungi are microscopic organisms that actually look like plants when seen under a microscope. Several different species of fungi may infect the feet. Most physicians now realize that so-called "athlete's foot" can be caused by the common tinea (ringworm) fungus, certain yeast-type fungi, or various types of bacteria.

Tinea infections of the feet differ in appearance. One infection may involve redness, cracking, and excessive softening of the toe webs along with itching and burning. Another may be characterized by a blistering eruption of the sole of the foot that either accompanies the common form of infection or appears alone.

Another fungal species produces a reddish or purplish color growth in the laboratory test tube and produces a much less inflamed, dry, scaling rash of the thick horny layer of the sole of the foot. This species also tends to induce infection of the nails and to cause an eruption of the top of the foot more often than the other species.

Another type of fungus is yeastlike, creamy, very soft-looking and has the same oyster-white color as yeast. The yeast-like fungus tends to infect only toe webs and toenails. The webs are moist, red, and split.

Of course, not all red, itchy rashes on the feet are "athlete's foot." Other skin diseases such as psoriasis, eczema, and allergic skin reactions may produce scaling, itching and redness indistinguishable from athlete's foot. Thus, the diagnosis of "athlete's foot" may be complicated.

TREATMENT OF ATHLETE'S FOOT

What is the best treatment for athlete's foot?
Treatment of athlete's foot depends on the character and stage of eruption and the type of fungus responsible for the infection.

Acutely inflamed, blistering, and oozing conditions are best treated with soothing, antiseptic, and astringent wet dressings and bland pastes or ointments. When acute inflammation and blistering have subsided and it is certain that a fungal infection is present, specific antifungal remedies may be considered for application to the skin. Physicians may also prescribe internal agents when their use is indicated.

Treatment should be appropriate to the type of fungus. Treatment for the moldlike tinea fungus is quite different from that for the yeastlike fungus.

Self-medication can produce complications and prolong discomfort and disability, so it is best to consult a physician for diagnosis and treatment. Relief may be obtained through the use of simple and bland substances, but a specific approach to treatment will often require the attention of a physician who will make the necessary examination for confirmation of the diagnosis.

PREVENTION OF ATHLETE'S FOOT

What is the best way to prevent athlete's foot?
The presence of warm, moist skin encourages the growth of all types of fungi. Thus, prevention of infections requires regular and meticulous foot hygiene. Thorough drying after bathing is essential, with gentle removal of moist debris between the toes.

The skin, especially in susceptible areas between the toes, should not be allowed to remain moist. Careful attention to shoes and socks and the materials of which they are made will prevent excessive moisture from sweating. Heavy socks, usually of wool, can increase the sweating of feet and induce infection. Other materials such as orlon, nylon, and dacron are both warming and occlusive, and should be avoided by people who have a tendency to sweat excessively as well as those in moist, humid climates. In such cases socks of 100 percent cotton are preferred. Rubber or synthetic shoe soles may also encourage too much warmth and moisture. Wear sandals or aerated shoes during warm weather. After participating in sports such as tennis, golf, or jogging, remove shoes and socks as soon as possible and shower or at least wash your feet. Those who work in hot, humid climates or must wear heavy, occlusive work shoes, such as steelworkers, construction workers, miners, and launderers, should also follow this procedure.

Medications, applied in treatment, can also collect moisture in the webs and should be avoided. Foot powders applied too heavily tend to cake and produce irritation. Greasy preparations, such as ointments, tend to heat and excessively soften the skin.

18

Perspiration and Body Odor

CONTROL OF BODY ODOR

Please explain the cause of body odor and exactly what deodorants and antiperspirants do. Are these products alike?

The following summary will attempt to answer the several aspects of this question:

Body odor is commonly related to perspiration. Perspiration itself is essentially odorless; odor develops from the action of bacteria on secretions from the skin's glands. These bacteria are present on everyone's skin and are most active in warm, moist surroundings. For this reason body odors are likely to develop in areas of the body from which perspiration cannot evaporate readily; this is a special problem in hot and very humid weather.

Sweat is composed of the free-flowing liquid of the eccrine glands and the milky secretion of the apocrine glands. Eccrine sweat glands are widely distributed over the body surface, with some concentration on the forehead, palms, and soles. Heat or nervous tension stimulates them to produce large amounts of sweat. As this evaporates, the body is cooled. Eccrine sweat, which is brought about by heat alone, does not usually cause an odor problem.

Body odor is more apt to occur in times of emotional

stress, when apocrine as well as eccrine sweat is secreted. Functioning apocrine sweat glands are found mainly in the axillae (underarms), and the growth of the apocrines, which are closely associated with hair follicles, is stimulated by the same hormones that cause hair growth in the axillae. Secretion of these hormones begins at puberty and gradually decreases with advancing age. Hence, body odor is rarely a problem in children and old people.

The most effective way to control both bacterial growth on the skin and body odor is by personal cleanliness. Bathing is a primary method of controlling body odor, and clothing, which also collects odors and bacteria, should be changed daily as well as cleaned or laundered frequently.

Deodorants are products formulated to mask or diminish body odor. Various chemicals may be incorporated into the preparations to perform this function. Deodorants, however, do not in any way affect the production or flow of perspiration.

Antiperspirants, as the name indicates, incorporate chemicals intended to reduce the amount of perspiration that reaches the skin's surface. They usually also have a deodorant effect. Deodorants and antiperspirants are discussed in the chapter "Other Cosmetic Products."

EXCESSIVE PERSPIRATION

I perspire excessively. What do you advise?
It is important to realize that perspiration is not under voluntary control. Many emotional and environmental factors other than heat influence the quantity of perspiration. Excessive sweating may be related to low-grade infections, internal disorders, other medical problems, or menopause.

Most antiperspirants contain some type of aluminum salt that temporarily reduces the delivery of perspiration to the skin surface. None will completely stop perspiration—nor is this desirable, because excessive local dryness would result. The efficiency of such antiperspirants is limited: often a few hours of control is followed by a rebound phenomenon, so that increased perspiration occurs as the effectiveness of the agent wears off. (See Chapter 3, "Other Cosmetic Products," for additional information on antiperspirants.)

In severe cases, drugs given orally under a physician's care may control excessive sweating, but undesirable side-effects may limit their effectiveness. Some of these drugs also appear to be effective when applied topically to the skin; however, this use is still experimental.

The following suggestions may be helpful in dealing with excessive perspiration: (1) Be sure the product you purchase is labeled as an antiperspirant, since many useful deodorants are not intended to have, and do not possess, antiperspirant activity. (2) Explore several products; some may be more effective than others. (3) Consult a physician regarding possible underlying medical causes of excessive sweating and any benefit that might be gained from the use of oral or topical drugs. (4) Adjust to the physiological problems by learning to protect clothing, with, for example, dress shields.

CONTROLLING SWEATY PALMS

What can I do to control excessive sweating of the palms? It's embarrassing when I am at parties and other social functions.

The palms, along with soles and forehead, have greater concentrations of sweat glands than most other areas of the body and are common sites for localized excessive sweating (hyperhidrosis). This condition is common and occurs in "normal" individuals; some people simply sweat more than others, and some have sweat glands that require less stimulation to make them active. Such sweating can occur in youngsters as well as in adults. Hyperhidrosis may be a real problem when it becomes severe enough to interfere with work or social life.

Emotional stress usually plays a greater role than thermal

stimulation in excessive sweating of the palms; thus, the problem is more acute on important occasions associated with tension—when you want to look your best. At such times, try to remain as "cool, calm, and collected" as possible. Avoiding caffeine-containing beverages such as coffee, which are stimulants, may help.

Unfortunately, no completely effective medical treatment for this condition is available. The benefits that can be expected from any therapy are limited and choice of treatment depends on many factors: the degree of hyperhidrosis, responsiveness to available measures, complications such as skin disorders, allergic sensitivity to ingredients in topical treatments, or potential side-effects of internal treatments. Physicians can prescribe various topical preparations that are helpful for moderate hyperhidrosis.

Sedatives or tranquilizers may be prescribed for severe cases on important occasions. Other systemic drugs are usually reserved for patients in whom the disorder presents a significant social or occupational handicap.

Occasionally the only successful treatment for severe palmar hyperhidrosis is cervical sympathectomy, an operation that involves excision of the nerves associated with sweating of the palms. Your physician will advise you about treatment for your particular case.

SEVERE PERSPIRATION PROBLEM

I perspire a great deal. Is there an antiperspirant that will keep my underarms completely dry?
No antiperspirant product will keep your underarms completely dry, especially during physical activity. The best that can be hoped for is that it will decrease perspiration flow. To stop perspiration completely, sweat ducts must be blocked—and this is not desirable. While products could be formulated to cause more complete blockage, these might produce a high incidence of skin reactions, discomfort, and other problems.

The first step in controlling underarm perspiration is to limit your physical activity. The second is to provide for easier evaporation of perspiration by wearing loose, porous clothing and dehumidifying your environment. If you can't do either of these, look for assistance from cosmetic products such as antiperspirants. (For more information on antiperspirants, see Chapter 3, "Other Cosmetic Products.")

Women can deal with excessive perspiration by wearing dress shields made of a material such as cotton that absorbs perspiration from the skin and a waterproof shield to protect clothes from moisture.

CONTROLLING UNDERARM ODOR

What can be done to prevent underarm perspiration odor? I have used all brands of cream, roll-on, and spray deodorants, only to find that within a couple of hours they are no longer effective. What causes this?

The primary cause of unpleasant underarm odor is the action of skin bacteria on secretions of the apocrine sweat glands, which are especially abundant in this area.

Cleanliness is the most important means of controlling such body odor. Removing underarm hair helps reduce the number of bacteria present. Clothes also may collect odors, so it is important to wear clean clothes and discard those that have acquired persistent odors or appear to be associated with odor problems. Deodorants provide some help in dealing with the odor problem, but do not replace cleanliness.

If you are careful to keep your body and clothes clean, are using a deodorant, and still have body odor, it may be due to some other factor such as certain metabolic and infectious diseases, some drugs, and foods such as garlic, onions, and asparagus. If you believe your odor is unusual, discuss the problem with your physician.

"FEMININE" ODOR AND DEODORANTS

What causes odor in the vaginal area?

A certain degree of distinctive odor is normal in the vaginal area, although Americans (shaped by advertising) tend to regard all odors—even normal ones—as undesirable. A traditional and effective method of combating odor here, as elsewhere on the body, is cleanliness—regular soap-and-water cleansing as part of the normal shower or tub bath is all that most people require to combat odor.

"Body odor" is caused by bacteria acting on perspiration, mucus, and sebum (oil) present on skin, hair, and sometimes even clothes. This may be a special problem on body areas that are normally warm and moist. For women who feel they may have a special odor problem, feminine deodorant sprays can supplement but not replace cleanliness. However, feminine deodorant sprays have no medical usefulness and are potentially harmful.

If significant vaginal discharge and/or odor are present, consult your physician to find the cause.

What are feminine deodorant sprays? How safe and effective are they?

Feminine deodorant sprays are aerosols for application to a woman's external genital area. Most consist of an emollient or powder of the type used in cosmetics, perfume, and a propellant; a few contain antibacterial agents. They act much as underarm deodorants do to inhibit bacterial growth and reduce the possibility of offensive odor.

The major brands of feminine deodorant sprays were carefully formulated and tested so that the incidence of allergic reactions would be minimal. However, some women experience irritation or allergic reactions from using the products. Some physicians report an increased incidence of local reactions among patients who use them. These reactions have consisted of itching, burning, and blisters in the area sprayed.

*Why can't underarm deodorants be used for this purpose
if they are similar to feminine deodorants?*

Antiperspirants and deodorants are not the same thing. Most
antiperspirants and some underarm deodorants contain aluminum salts, which are very irritating to mucous membrane
tissue. Deodorants specifically formulated for the external genital area do not contain ingredients known to cause such irritation.

*How should these products be used? Should any special
precautions be observed?*

Feminine deodorant sprays are designed for application to the
external genital area only. They should not be sprayed into the
vagina. The container should be held at least 8 inches from
the skin. Feminine deodorant sprays should not be applied to
broken, irritated, or itching skin. If a rash, irritation, an unusual vaginal discharge or discomfort develops, use of the spray
should be discontinued immediately and your physician should
be consulted.

Some women use these sprays daily, but a large number
use them only during the menstrual period. They may be
sprayed on the skin, but should not be sprayed on sanitary
pads or tampons. Feminine deodorant sprays should not be
used directly before or after sexual intercourse—a number of
cases of genital irritation in both men and women have been
reported from misuse of these preparations.

*Is vaginal douching necessary to maintain cleanliness of
the normal vagina?*

Most gynecologists agree that in the absence of vaginal infections or specific medical indications, daily douching is not only
unnecessary but unwise.

Douching of the normal vagina can lead to pathological
conditions. Strong chemicals and changes in the normal bacterial flora and acid medium can injure cells in the lining of
the vagina. Excess unnecessary douching can itself lead to
the production of a discharge.

Many women try to eliminate the discharge by increased douching, but only succeed in aggravating the condition initiated by the douching.

YELLOW PERSPIRATION ON CLOTHES

My bras, dress shields, slips, and blouses are discolored with a yellow stain that I can't remove. Could perspiration be the cause? What can I do to prevent the discoloration? Staining of clothing in the underarm area can be caused by secretion of colored sweat from the body, by discoloration of sweat after it reaches the skin surface, or by some material that comes in contact with the skin in this area.

Secretion of yellow sweat from the body (chromhidrosis) is very rare, although it may occur. The apocrine sweat glands, which are active only in the underarm area and are responsible for body odor, may secrete a yellowish sweat, and some drugs may cause sweat to turn yellow. However, colored sweat is most often due to some external matter that comes in contact with the skin and either interacts with the sweat to turn it yellow or, by itself, stains the skin and/or clothing.

Sweat that is colorless may turn yellow on interacting with a variety of organisms on the skin, either bacteria or fungi. Chemicals in cosmetics, antiperspirants, and fabrics may also interact with sweat to produce a yellowish discoloration.

Carefully evaluate everything that comes in contact with your underarms as a possible cause. Does the discoloration appear on all types of fabrics—cottons, synthetics, and treated fabrics (permanent press)—or only on certain types of clothing? If discoloration appears on all types of fabrics, it may be due to ingredients in antiperspirants or cosmetic preparations (lotions and powders, for instance) applied to your underarms.

Some people react to common ingredients in deodorants and antiperspirants, such as perfumes, by developing a yellowish stain in the underarm area of dress shields, slips, bras, and white or pastel clothing after only a few wearings. Changing to a deodorant or an antiperspirant that claims to be unscented may help to avoid this problem. Stains already present in clothing can be removed by use of prelaundry cleaning preparations. At least one popular antiperspirant now advertises its nonstaining quality because of the perfume it contains and a special ingredient added to the formulation to aid in removal of stains during the washing process.

You can determine whether your antiperspirant is the cause of the discoloration by wearing a set of new, unstained underclothes and outer clothes at the time that you are using a new antiperspirant; if the fabrics do not become stained, you may have found the solution to your problem. If the staining continues, you will have to investigate other things that come in contact with your underarms.

If all the above efforts fail, you may want to consult a dermatologist to determine whether your condition is due to bacterial or fungal infection, drugs, or other medical problems; in such a case, control of the underlying cause will control the yellow staining.

19

Soaps and Bathing

TOILET SOAPS

Are some toilet soaps less drying than others?
The mechanism by which soap and water washing may dry
the skin is not well understood. Soap and water cleansing
removes most substances from the skin surface including con-
taminants such as dirt, oily soils, and bacteria, and some
natural skin products—oils, dead cells, and sweat. Too frequent washing may also remove substances that normally keep
the skin soft and pliable by holding a small amount of water
within its layers.

On the whole, there is probably little difference, if any,
in drying effects of various types and brands of toilet soap.
No well-substantiated evidence demonstrates that the addition of neutral fats or cold cream will counteract the drying
effect of soaps. And it is hardly likely that a cleansing agent,
such as soap, can accomplish two diametrically opposed tasks
in a single washing operation: (1) removal of soil from the
skin, and (2) deposition of a fat or cream on the skin.

Where dryness does occur, emollient creams should be
used.

TRANSPARENT SOAPS

What is the difference between transparent soap bars and regular soap bars? What kind of soap is better for sensitive skin?

Transparent soap bars (or glycerin soaps, as they are sometimes called) have been available for many years. Because they are more costly and time consuming to manufacture, and therefore more expensive, their market has been small.

Transparent soap bars differ from opaque soap in the combination of ingredients and in the method of manufacture.

Opaque soap is usually prepared from a mixture of tallow and a lesser proportion of an oil such as coconut or olive oil. In transparent soap, the fat content is increased by including some castor oil and/or resin. During the manufacture of transparent soap, other ingredients such as alcohol, glycerin, and sugar are added to produce bars that are transparent and of a softer consistency.

Regular toilet soap bars, called milled soap, are compressed by machinery and extruded as a continuous bar. Transparent soap, in the traditional method of manufacture, is prepared in batches and solidified in frames or molds. Often transparent soap cakes must be stored for several weeks to harden and develop full translucency before they can be shipped. Today, however, it is possible to make transparent soap bars comparable in quality and price to opaque milled soap using conventional soap-making equipment, so that people are offered a wider selection of brands at more economical prices.

Since transparent soaps are softer and more soluble in water than milled toilet bars, they do not last or lather as well. On the other hand, many transparent soaps claim to be "neutral," and less drying or irritating to the skin than milled toilet bars, which are generally slightly alkaline. Transparent bars are advertised as more acceptable for people with skin problems. However, such evaluations are more subjective than objective. The choice of one type of soap over another depends primarily on personal preference, unless a skin problem exists for which a physician has recommended a particular type of soap.

In addition to transparent soaps and opaque soaps, there are superfatted soaps, "cold cream" soaps, antibacterial soaps, abrasive soaps, and "soap" bars that incorporate synthetic detergents instead of soap. In some cases, scent may influence a buyer's choice as much as the effects of the soap on the skin.

DIFFERENCES BETWEEN SOAPS AND DETERGENTS

What is the difference between soaps and detergents especially with respect to their effects on the skin?
While they differ somewhat chemically as well as in their tendency to form "hard-water scum," soaps and detergents are both active and useful cleansing agents.

Soaps are made from animal and vegetable fats. In use, they combine with the minerals of hard water (chiefly calcium and magnesium salts) to form an unattractive and insoluble scum or curd on skin, bathtubs, and fabrics.

Synthetic detergents, most of which are made of petroleum derivatives, vary greatly in chemical composition and range from extremely mild to moderately irritating to the skin. Most detergents on the market today, however, are said to be equivalent in mildness to the soap products used for the same purpose. A major advantage of synthetic detergents is that they do not deposit a hard-water scum.

HOW TO DISTINGUISH BETWEEN SOAPS AND DETERGENTS

How can the consumer distinguish between soaps and detergents?
The consumer must rely on label information to make this

distinction. However, there is no standard statement, consistent from product to product, that indicates clearly the nature of the contents. Most soap products carry the word "soap" with reasonable prominence, and most synthetic detergents have some reference to "no soap scum" or a similar distinction. The necessary information is almost always on the carton, but the exact words and their location (sometimes in the trademark statement) may vary considerably.

SOAP IS SOAP

What's the difference between a "deodorant" soap and an "antibacterial" soap?

Basically, there is little difference between the two. Bacteria act on perspiration and other skin debris, causing body odor. Since any soap cleanses the skin, it can be considered a deodorant soap. However, "deodorant" soap marketed as such usually contains a perfume to mask undesirable odors or an antibacterial agent that inhibits the growth of odor-producing bacteria.

An "antibacterial" soap contains one or more chemical agents designed to inhibit the growth of bacteria.

REACTIONS FROM CHANGE IN DETERGENT

I have developed a rash on my hands that began after the formula of my regular household detergent was apparently changed. Could the rash have been caused by this product, which I have used satisfactorily for years?

The formulas for detergent products change frequently. The manufacturers usually inform us in TV commercials and advertisements that such changes improve the cleansing or brightening effect.

Skin can become irritated by a new formulation even though past experience with the same brand was satisfactory.

The simplest solution is to switch brands until you find a product less irritating to your hands that does the cleaning job you expect. In some cases the skin reaction may not be related to the detergent at all.

Often hands that have been irritated by contact with water and detergents, or from other causes, do not heal readily of their own accord. If the dermatitis persists, consult your physician to check for other aggravating factors and for suitable treatment.

ENZYME DETERGENTS AND PRESOAKS

What are enzyme presoaks and laundry detergents? Are they more irritating to the skin than conventional detergents?

Enzyme presoaks and detergents represent another development in the formulation of laundry products. Detergents containing enzyme ingredients are used in the same manner as conventional detergents, while enzyme presoak products are used in a soaking step before the regular washing cycle.

Enzymes are special catalysts found in all living systems—animal, plant, or microbial. They are responsible for complex biochemical reactions of life processes. Various enzymes are used in many industrial processes, for example baking, cheese-making, and brewing. Others are found in meat tenderizing products. Enzymes used in enzyme detergents are produced by microorganisms. While the enzymes themselves are not living organisms, special care must be taken in processing to separate them from the organisms that produced them.

Enzymes in detergent and presoak products are selected for their ability to function under laundering conditions. These enzyme preparations certainly aren't the magical products that TV commercials imply; however, they do seem to remove many organic stains such as blood, feces, grass, gravy, and juice from fabrics better than conventional detergents—

particularly when such stains have become fixed, for example, by heat treatment. Effects on other stains and soils are about the same for both types of products.

Enzyme products appear to be especially effective as presoaks. Enzyme activity is used up quickly during washing and is easily blocked by chlorine bleaches. Therefore, chlorine and enzyme products should not be used at the same time.

Manufacturers claim that enzyme laundry products were tested extensively on animals and humans before being released for consumer use. Tests on human volunteers showed that enzyme washing products were essentially equivalent in their effects on the skin to conventional products. This was true for the wearing of clothing washed in the products as well as for direct contact with the products.

Manufacturers also claim that they have been attentive to customer comments about these products since marketing. They report that only an occasional person finds enzyme products more irritating than the detergent used previously. On the other hand, some consumers and physicians insist that they produce more skin reactions than conventional detergents. The truth probably lies somewhere in between. A new product is often blamed—sometimes erroneously—for adverse skin reactions because it is the first factor that occurs to the affected person. While enzyme products are undoubtedly responsible for some reactions, they do not appear to present a significant hazard to the skin.

BATH PREPARATIONS

How do bubble bath preparations and bath salts or crystals compare? Are any hazards associated with their use? Originally, bubble bath preparations were designed to provide fragrance and bubbles or foam. Bath salts or crystals provided fragrances while softening water. Today's bath preparations, however, are usually combination products that perform several functions; for instance, a bubble bath preparation may contain a water softener and a bath oil in addition to bubble ingredients and fragrance.

Bath salts present a potential hazard because they sometimes make water too alkaline, causing itching or redness, especially to sensitive skin.

Bubble bath preparations should be well mixed with water before the user sits down in the tub. This is particularly important for children, since physicians have reported urinary tract irritations in youngsters resulting from contact with concentrated bubble bath solutions. Children may also develop dry and irritated skin from excessive bathing.

CHILDREN'S BUBBLE BATH PREPARATIONS

My children are perfectly normal—they hate to take baths. But if I put bubble bath into the tub, I have an easier time urging the kids to get into it. Recently, however, I read that some bubble baths might be dangerous. How can I know which products are safe for my children to use? Bubble bath products on the market now are safe when used properly.

There has been some concern about children's bubble bath preparations because a few reports from physicians and parents in recent years have associated bubble bath products with urinary tract irritation in small children, especially girls. No one knows for sure what caused the irritation, but a few of the detergents used in the products were thought to be responsible.

At the request of the Federal Food and Drug Administration, the two companies that used these detergents have reformulated their products. However, since all detergents can irritate delicate tissues, this does not mean that the new bubble baths—or any bubble bath—can be used without proper precautions.

Scientists think that irritation can occur whenever the skin or mucous membranes are exposed to a concentrated solution of bubble bath preparation, which can happen if the bubble bath is not thoroughly mixed with enough water before the child gets into the tub.

Don't let your child pour half the bottle of bubble bath into the tub. You measure out the amount that is recommended on the package—no more—and make sure it is thoroughly mixed with enough water before the child gets in. If you do this and irritation still occurs, stop using the bubble bath for a while. If the irritation goes away, then the bubble bath probably caused it and you should stop using it (but you can try another brand). If it doesn't go away, you probably should take your child to a doctor.

SOAP VS. CREAM FOR FACIAL CLEANSING

I have been told that I should never wash my face with soap and water—that I should use a cleansing cream instead. Is this true? Is soap and water cleansing bad for the complexion?

Regular cleansing of the skin is certainly desirable for cosmetic and esthetic reasons, whether or not it is important as a matter of health. Cleansing removes sebum (oily secretion), sweat, skin debris, dirt, cosmetics, and a certain number of bacteria and can be carried out most quickly and effectively with water and a mild soap or detergent.

Normal as well as oily skin easily tolerates this treatment on a regular basis. If your facial skin is exceptionally dry, a lotion or cream may be helpful. Under these conditions, and especially when the temperature and humidity are both low, cleansing with a cream, alternated with soap and water washing, may be more comfortable. (Cleansing creams are discussed in Chapter 1.)

THE BEST WAY TO CLEANSE THE SKIN

What is the best way to cleanse the skin?
There is no one way of cleansing the skin that is best for everyone. Climate, work and recreational activities, availability of facilities, individual tastes, age, and health all influence skin cleansing. Many people in the United States probably bathe too often for really good skin care. Bathing once a day is adequate and may even, during the winter months or for elderly people, be too much of a good thing.

General rules for cleansing the skin include: (1) Avoid using very hot water and scrubbing with strong soaps; these cause excessive degreasing of the skin and subsequent dryness, chapping, and itching. (2) Don't massage soap into your skin unless advised to do so by your physician for a specific reason. (3) Don't use medicated soaps unless advised to do so by your physician. (4) Use sufficient water to rinse away all traces of soap. (5) Cleanse your face with soap and water instead of with cleansing cream if your skin is oily; alternate between soap and water and cleansing cream if your skin is excessively dry. (6) Avoid too frequent bathing, especially in winter; this can cause your skin to become dry, red, and irritated.

EFFECTS OF HARD AND SOFT WATER ON SKIN, HAIR, AND SCALP

Is soft water better for my hair and skin than hard water?
Yes. The salts and minerals (calcium and magnesium) in hard water interact with soap to form an insoluble residue that is difficult to rinse away. The remaining soap can cause irritation and itching of your skin.

If hard water is a problem in your area, use synthetic detergents instead of soap whenever possible. These produce little or no residue.

Soft water is also important to hair care. When hair is

washed with soap and hard water, the residue clings to both scalp and hair, dulling the hair's natural luster. It also interferes with waving and coloring procedures since clean hair, without residue, is essential for uniform application of permanent wave solutions, setting solutions and hair coloring preparations. Most shampoos today are partly or completely detergents instead of soap.

BATH OILS AND DRY SKIN

Are bath oils of any value in controlling dry skin symptoms?

Bath oils help to control dry skin symptoms resulting from excessive bathing, the normal process of aging, and low humidity conditions encountered during colder seasons. However, lotions and creams applied directly to the skin are more effective in relieving these conditions; bath oils should be considered a supplement to other measures. Most bath oil deposited on the skin during bathing is wiped off by the towel when drying.

Bath oils aid in controlling "bath itch," a condition encountered particularly during the winter. But a word of caution is advisable in this regard: itching is a symptom of some internal disorders. If itching is general and persists, consult your physician to make sure that there is no underlying condition to be treated.

Many bath oils are available today and new ones are appearing regularly. Some float on top of the water; others disperse throughout it. A variety of oils and fragrances are employed, but it has never been clearly established that any particular type of bath oil is clearly superior to another.

One characteristic all bath oils share is that they may make the tub quite slippery. Everyone, particularly older people, should be aware of this and should be especially careful to avoid slipping and possible severe injury when a bath oil is used.

The mounting of holding rails in the bathtub area is a worthwhile precaution.

PEARLS AND BATH OIL

I was given bath oil "pearls" as a present. I haven't used them because I always thought liquid bath oil did more for skin. Is there a difference?

Yes, but not much. The chief difference is the obvious physical form. The degree of fragrance may also differ, but the effects on skin are essentially the same.

Bath oil capsules consist of small amounts of bath oil enclosed in soft, flexible, gelatin capsules that dissolve in hot water. The bath oil may be colored, or the capsules themselves may appear "pearly" due to pigmentation, such as mica particles coated with titanium dioxide.

The perfume content, often 10 percent or more, is usually higher in bath oil capsules than in liquid bath oil. A single large capsule may yield a noticeable fragrance. Two or three of the small, pearl-sized capsules may be needed to perfume a bath. If fragrance is what you seek, you may prefer capsules to liquid bath oil.

Effects of bath oils on the skin are discussed in the previous exchange.

20

Sunlight and the Skin

TANNING WITHOUT BURNING

What is the quickest and safest way to get a good suntan? I usually end up getting a painful sunburn instead.

Every year as summer approaches people head for beaches, parks, backyards, swimming pools—wherever the sun shines brightly—to roast their exposed skin for the sake of a "beautiful tan."

Actually, the sun's beneficial effects are almost nil, and you should consider the adverse effects before joining the sun worshipers this summer. Excessive sun exposure permanently damages the skin and leads to premature aging, wrinkling, leathery texture, and precancerous and cancerous skin conditions. The only beneficial effect of tanning, aside from the psychological feeling of well-being, is the formation of vitamin D—which the normal American diet provides amply. If you insist on getting a tan, however, several pointers can help minimize burning:

First, you must realize that you can't bake all day in the sun for one weekend and end up with a tan. A suntan should be acquired gradually.

Skin varies greatly in the amount of sun it can tolerate. Dark-skinned, dark-haired, dark-eyed individuals generally have more tolerance to sunlight than redheads, blonds, and fair-skinned individuals. You must learn for yourself how much sun you can tolerate.

For most people with light skin, first exposure to the sun early in the season should not exceed 15 or 20 minutes for each side—back and face. If you begin tanning later in the season, the first exposure should be even shorter, particularly if you begin in a vacation climate sunnier than the one in which you live. Sudden change in sun intensity eliminates the protection that develops with a gradual increase of sunlight in a given location.

You can increase exposure time by about one-third each day. After about 4 days new pigment should begin to darken your skin; after a week there should be enough skin thickening and pigment (tan) to provide added protection against burning. These statements do not apply to freckled, red-haired persons, who must be more careful.

The time of day is also important. The sun's burning rays are most intense between 11 A.M. and 3 P.M. No sunburn is likely before 8 A.M. or after 4 P.M.

Rays reflected from sand and water can burn even if there is no direct exposure; you can get a burn while sitting on the beach under an umbrella. Rays reflected from snow increase sunburn potential for skiers.

Don't be fooled by hazy or foggy, overcast days. These atmospheric conditions scatter the sun's burning rays and can produce severe sunburn.

Suntan preparations are of limited value. Most commercially available suntan lotions contain chemicals, called sunscreens, that absorb specific wavelengths of the burning ultraviolet rays of sunlight to various degrees. The more effective lotions allow you to stay in the sun longer with less risk of burning. They do not shut out all radiation, or you would never tan. Among the most effective sunscreens are the salicylates, the newer benzophenone compounds, and para-aminobenzoic acid and its derivatives. Before purchasing a suntan product, read the label for the sunscreen ingredient, which is usually listed, or check the brand-name guide to sun products at the end of this chapter. Suntan products must be reapplied at least every 2 hours, after each swim, and whenever the protective film may have rubbed off or washed away.

Skin care following sunbathing is important to help offset the sun's drying effect. Apply an emollient lotion or cream to your skin after bathing and before retiring.

If you get a sunburn in spite of precautions, apply a soothing lotion or ointment such as cold cream or baby lotion; apply wet compresses, or soak in a tub of plain water to relieve the pain. However, a word of caution about the use of commercial sunburn preparations: these products contain ingredients that may cause allergic skin reactions. If pain is excessive or extensive blistering appears, consult a physician.

PROTECTION FROM THE SUN

How can I protect my skin from overexposure to the sun and still enjoy outdoor sports this summer?
Your skin cannot be completely protected from the sun, but you can take several measures to minimize overexposure and subsequent damage.

A sunshade preparation containing opaque chemicals such as zinc oxide or titanium dioxide provides the most protection by preventing the sun's ultraviolet rays from reaching your skin. Clothing that is not too porous offers similar protection.

Sunblocking preparations containing chemical sunscreens to lessen the degree of burning and tanning give varying amounts of protection, but none is 100 percent effective. In addition, they are partially removed by swimming, perspiring, or contact with clothing and must be reapplied fairly frequently.

Sunscreen and tanning preparations that claim to minimize burning and at the same time promote a tan are of less value than sunblocks, since tanning can also damage skin. Makeup preparations containing sunscreens are even farther down on the protective scale. They offer minimum defense against tanning or a sunburn.

The alternative to using one of these preparations is reducing or eliminating your time in the sun during the hours when its ultraviolet, or burning, rays are strongest—from 11 until 3. No sunburn is likely before 8 A.M. or after 4 P.M.

SKIN THAT BURNS EASILY

When my friend and I go to the beach for a day, she ends up with a tan while I get a painful burn but never a tan. What can I do to obtain a nice dark tan like hers?

As explained in a previous answer, the ease with which people tan or burn depends to a large extent on the amount of pigment in their skin, i.e., their skin color. If your friend tans readily, she probably has a darker complexion than you and therefore has more pigment on her skin surface to darken and produce a tanned effect.

People with fair-colored skin (redheads and blonds) may be able to acquire some tan and avoid serious burning by repeated small doses of exposure to sunlight. On the other hand, light-colored skin usually is unable to produce enough protective pigment to avoid burning. So it is advisable to cut down on sun exposure by remaining covered and using sunscreen preparations. Skin damage (aging skin and small skin growths) tends to appear early in life among light-skinned people who expose themselves excessively to the sun.

SUNBURNED LIPS

On my vacation several people, including myself, developed sunburn on the lower lip. What causes it, and what can be done to heal it?

This phenomenon occurs most frequently in fair-skinned people and those who have protruding lips or breathe through their mouths much of the time, thus keeping their lips parted. Either situation allows considerable sunlight exposure to unprotected lips.

Prevention is the most important consideration. Lipstick provides significant protection for women. Otherwise, women as well as men should wear a topical sunscreen. Several preparations are specifically designed for this purpose, some in the form of colorless lipstick.

Sunburned lips should be treated with a cool, wet compress or a bland ointment. Medical treatment is advisable if the reaction is severe.

REACTION FROM WINTER SUN VACATION

Two years ago, I went south for the winter and got prickly heat. Last year it was sunburn. What can I do to avoid these problems this year?

Prickly heat, a red, itchy eruption, is caused by temporary blockage of the sweat glands. Profuse sweating and thick coats of suntan oil can aggravate the condition. Sunburn, the other winter vacation menace, occurs if you don't protect your skin properly or if you stay in the sun too long.

Practicing "sense in the sun" can help you avoid both problems. Give your body time to adjust to the hot, usually humid climate and intense sun. Avoid heavy, greasy suntan preparations—excellent suntan and sunblock agents are available that are relatively greaseless. Regulate your sun exposure. The sun in the south is much more intense than it is in northern areas, so you will burn faster. Don't sunbathe at midday when the sun's rays are most intense, and, if you start to sweat profusely, get out of the sun and cool off.

SUN POISONING

I'd like to know how long a person has to stay out of the sun after a case of sun poisoning. I had a severe sunburn last year, and afterward was unable to go out in the sun all summer. Every time I did, I broke out and my skin itched constantly.

"Sun poisoning" is a lay term used for a variety of acute and chronic responses to the sun's rays. Your description suggests a type of sensitivity, probably an "allergy," to the sun. These responses depend primarily on sunburn rays that do not pass through window glass. Such reactions are usually chronic and reappear indefinitely with further sun exposure. However, in many patients the reaction disappears spontaneously within two or three years.

The problem frequently begins after a severe sunburn response. As with other allergies, the best treatment is to avoid the causative agent. Though some patients do develop protection by gradual reexposure, most find that they must avoid the sun's rays with protective clothing (wide-brimmed hats and the like), physical barriers, or sunblocking agents, and at times internal medications prescribed by a physician. Sunblocks should be applied frequently, especially if the patient is swimming, perspiring, or otherwise rubbing off the material, and midday spring and summer sun should be avoided, since the rays are more intense at these times.

Occasionally sunlight sensitivity is due to skin contact with photosensitizers (ingredients in certain plants, cosmetics, skin lotions, and even sunscreen preparations) or the use of certain internal medications. In such cases, further reactions are usually, though not always, prevented by eliminating the photosensitizer. Since these problems are frequently quite disturbing and persistent, it usually is necessary to consult a physician for proper diagnosis and treatment.

PHOTOSENSITIVE SKIN

Please explain the cause and treatment of photosensitive skin. My husband has had this condition for 3½ years. Treatment by several physicians, including specialists, has not been successful.

Photosensitive skin exhibits an exaggerated response or sensitivity to light. The prerequisite is the presence of a photosensitizing agent in the skin, followed by exposure to light. Natural sunlight is usually the source of light that produces photosensitivity reactions both indoors and outdoors. Common window glass does not filter out the rays of the sun responsible for some photosensitivity reactions. In addition, some artificial light sources, among them fluorescent tubes, can cause reactions.

The skin reaction may consist of redness, itching, inflammation, and rash. Some photosensitizers also produce discoloration or areas of hyperpigmentation (brown spots).

Numerous agents found in an enormous number and variety of items can act as photosensitizers. The list includes certain medications and foods, and a variety of items that come in contact with the skin. Commonly used products that may contain photosensitizers include perfumes, antibacterial soaps, synthetic detergents, medicated cosmetics, shampoos, antiseptic creams, hair conditioners, after-shave products, and other men's fragrance products.

Because of the variety of agents that may produce photosensitivity it is sometimes very difficult, if not impossible, for a physician to determine the cause of a patient's reaction.

Even if the photosensitizing agent is identified, it may be impossible for the patient to avoid further contact with it, since the agent may be present in several different products with which the patient comes in contact.

Until recently, identification of potentially harmful products was frequently impossible because ingredient information often did not appear on product labels, or appeared in the form of imaginative but uninformative designations (each manufacturer had his own special code name for the same ingredient). Although many manufacturers are still reluctant to divulge ingredient information, fortunately the present tendency in the consumer product area is toward universal, more informative ingredient labeling.

Once sensitization to one agent has occurred, a person may also become sensitized to closely related chemicals. If the photosensitizing agent is identified and further contact avoided, the skin condition usually improves rapidly. Unfortunately, in a few people the condition does not improve and may persist for months or years after the last known exposure.

As sunlight usually is the cause of photosensitive reactions, the photosensitive person should avoid or minimize exposure to sunlight. Protective clothing and sunscreen preparations can provide some protection when exposure is unavoidable. Commercial sunblocking preparations, ointments containing opaque chemicals such as zinc oxide and titanium dioxide, and prescription preparations may be used as sunscreens. None of these products is 100 percent effective, and degree and length of effectiveness vary. Some deposit a greasy and/or visible film on the skin that may be considered cosmetically undesirable.

SUNLIGHT AND SKIN CANCER

Can sunlight cause skin cancer? Do I have to worry about ordinary exposure?

Increasing evidence shows that the sun's ultraviolet rays are an important factor in producing certain types of skin cancer: (1) about 90 percent of skin cancer is found on exposed areas, principally the face; (2) skin cancer is rare in blacks, who are also less susceptible to sunburn; (3) in the United States, more skin cancer occurs in the southern states where there is also more sunshine.

There is some evidence that a single, severe overexposure

to the sun (one severe sunburn) may cause cancer in later years as well as scarring or pigmentary changes. Also, scientists are increasingly concerned that many years of ordinary exposure may be harmful. Long years of being outdoors—as in the case of a cowboy, an athlete, a sailor, or a sun worshiper—definitely predisposes a person to skin cancer from exposure to sunlight.

INDOOR/OUTDOOR SUNTAN

Many health clubs have "sunrooms" where the entire body is exposed to ultraviolet rays—for an overall tan, I imagine. Is this dangerous? How does it compare with regular outdoor sunbathing?

Repeated and prolonged exposure to sunlight (artificial or real) will eventually cause premature evidence of aging, such as dryness and wrinkling, as well as precancerous and cancerous conditions of the skin. Both sunlamps and the sun emit ultraviolet rays that cause these problems.

Whether you sunbathe indoors or out, don't try to get a tan in one day, and be extra careful with sunlamps. You cannot safely spend as much time under a sunlamp as you can in the sun or even in a sunroom, primarily because you are so close to the energy source. If you use a sunlamp at home, follow the manufacturer's instructions for length of exposure, distance of the lamp from your body, and use of eye protection devices. Be sure to give your eyes this added protection because exposure to artificial sunlight is potentially more hazardous for them. Never look directly at ultraviolet bulbs—this could cause permanent damage or blindness. Keep a safe distance from the light source. In a properly designed sunroom, there should be no possibility of patrons getting too close to the lamps. At home, read the instruction manual to find out how far you should stay from the lamp.

EFFECTS OF SUNLAMPS

I am considering using a sunlamp to maintain a year-round tan. Can sunlamps cause skin cancer? Are they safe for a fair-complexioned person whose skin is slightly dry and sensitive?

Occasional exposure to sunlamps does not appear harmful, but the amount of exposure required to maintain a year-round tan would probably be excessive, and the potential for skin cancer would be the same as discussed in the previous answer. Experience indicates that artificial sunlamps are somewhat less dangerous in this respect than is natural sunlight. However, special precautions must be taken in using a sunlamp to protect your eyes and to time exposures carefully.

The sun seems to have a drying effect on skin. Since your skin is already dry, regular use of emollient (softening or soothing) creams would be wise.

SUNTAN REMOVAL

I got a deep tan this summer, but now that fall will soon be here it is undesirable. Is there any way to bleach the tan?

There is no safe and effective way to remove a suntan. Bleaching preparations are generally ineffective, especially for large areas.

In time your skin will naturally "bleach out" as the tanned skin is replaced by normally light skin. In the meantime, a makeup base several shades lighter than your tanned skin may be helpful.

In the future, remember that the best approach to assure a normally light skin in the fall is to minimize tanning in summer and avoid a deep tan that can persist for months. In addition, such overexposure to the sun contributes greatly to premature aging of the skin. The person who prizes a "peaches-and-cream" complexion should think twice before sunbathing day after day in summer.

SUNBURNING AND SKIING

Why do skiers, particularly at high altitudes, sometimes get a worse sunburn than sunbathers? What methods of prevention do you recommend?

The burning effect of sunshine is due in large part to ultraviolet radiation that accompanies visible light. Ultraviolet wave lengths, which are shorter than those of visible light, are intense in outer space. However, they are partially scattered and filtered by the atmosphere as they pass through it, especially if particulate matter such as smoke or smog is present.

In higher altitudes, sunlight does not pass through so deep a layer of atmosphere. Less particulate matter is present, so the sunburning effect is more intense. Another important factor is that the skier's skin receives additional exposure from the reflected radiation bouncing off the snow cover.

Since overexposure to sunlight is, in general, injurious and hastens the aging of skin, it should be avoided. Protective clothing should be and usually is employed, except in the moderate temperatures of spring skiing.

A number of sunblocking agents are also helpful. They include preparations containing benzophenones and those consisting of adequate concentrations of para-aminobenzoic acid (PABA) in a cream or alcohol base, as well as physical barrier preparations that contain physical sunscreens such as zinc oxide and titanium dioxide. In general, protective agents must be applied frequently because perspiration, rubbing, and contact with snow will remove them.

RELIEF FROM SUNBURN PAIN

I love the sun—too much, I guess, because I can't resist staying out longer than I should. What is the best way to relieve the pain of sunburn? Are there any preparations I can use to keep my skin from peeling?

There is no specific treatment for sunburn, but ointments, wet compresses, soothing lotions, and soaking in a tub of plain water usually help relieve sunburn pain. A bland cold cream or lotion may soothe the affected area, making it feel better, but don't use drying "shake lotions" such as calamine lotion. Commercial sunburn preparations often contain local anesthetics that may produce allergic skin reactions and cause additional discomfort. If pain is excessive or blistering extensive, consult a physician.

Unfortunately, no preparation will prevent or retard the peeling that always follows a severe sunburn.

MINERAL OIL SUNTAN PREPARATIONS

Will mineral oil or baby oil mixed with iodine make as good a suntan preparation as those commercially available? Some of my friends say they get a better tan with this kind of preparation.

Mineral oil or baby oil, used alone or mixed with iodine, will not prevent sunburning or promote suntanning. Most commercially available suntan preparations contain chemicals called sunscreens, which absorb specific wavelengths of the sun's ultraviolet rays that are responsible for burning. Thus they allow you to stay in the sun longer with less risk of burning.

Mineral oil and baby oil do not contain sunscreens. The addition of iodine to the oil does nothing more than stain the skin. The only thing these oils provide is lubrication that will help to minimize the sun's drying effects. However, too much grease on the skin in the form of mineral oil, baby oil, or a heavy suntan oil, combined with perspiration and skin irritation from sun exposure, can produce an itchy skin rash and folliculitis (inflamed hair follicles). If you want some protection from sunburning, use a regular sunscreen preparation that is not too greasy.

Sunscreen preparations vary widely in effectiveness. Those with adequate concentrations of sunscreen agents are fairly effective, if used properly. Reapply the preparation at least every 2 hours, after each swim, and whenever the protective film may have rubbed off or washed away. Most commercial sunscreen preparations are formulated to permit tanning while minimizing burning. No sunscreen preparation will prevent sunburn if you stay out too long or if the preparation wears off.

ARTIFICIAL TANNING PREPARATIONS

Are preparations that artificially tan skin safe to use? Do they offer the same protection as a true tan?
In general, the chemical tanning preparations that contain dihydroxyacetone (DHA) are safe, providing the user is not allergic or sensitive to their ingredients; sensitivity would be revealed by irritation or a burning sensation after use.

Occasionally, with prolonged use, the skin can become dry and scaly. Rough skin, warts, and moles often pick up extra color from the chemical tanners, which does not harm them but may be considered undesirable. These preparations should not be used on sore or raw spots or areas of infection. Color will most likely not develop in these areas anyway.

More recently, preparations known as "bronzers" have become available. These cosmetic products, usually a gel, contain color pigments that impart a tan color to the skin. No chemical reactions occur between the "bronzer" and the skin. Soap and water can remove the tan color.

Unless "bronzers" and DHA products also contain a sunscreen (read the label), they offer no protection at all from the sun. The false sense of security given by the brownish skin color may lead to excessive exposure and sunburn. These preparations have the advantage of giving the skin a tanned appearance without the damage associated with sunlight exposure.

SUNBLOCK PREPARATIONS

Are there any products I can apply that will provide protection against the sun's damaging effects but will permit me to enjoy outdoor sports and perhaps obtain just a little suntan?

In recent years, several products have been marketed that will protect normal skin from most of the sun's damaging rays and thus permit reasonable exposure to the sun. Several of these products are claimed to provide almost complete blockage of ultraviolet (sunburning) rays, while others are reported to attenuate the intensity of sunlight's direct effects and therefore to reduce ultraviolet exposure. The products are for some unknown reason less effective for people with abnormal sensitivity or allergy to the sun.

Since no sunblock product is 100 percent effective in blocking out all of the sun's rays, in actual practice they will permit limited to extensive tanning. Don't depend on these products to provide complete protection from intensive sunlight or for extended exposure—such as all day. Also, the products need to be reapplied periodically, as the protective layer of sunscreen may be diluted or rubbed off by perspiration, etc. Examples of some of the sunblock products are provided in the brand-name guide to products at the end of this chapter.

If you are abnormally sensitive to the sun, consult your physician about products that may be helpful.

BRAND-NAME GUIDE TO
SUN PREPARATIONS *

	Sunscreens (Permit tanning, minimum protection)	Sun Blocks (minimize tanning, intermediate to good burn protection)	Physical Barriers (Maximum burn protection)	Artificial Tanners (Dihydroxyacetone type, no burn protection unless sunscreen included)	Temporary Stains (No burn protection—wash off)	Lubricating Moisturizing Agents (No burn protection—minimize skin dryness)
Avon Sun Safe	•					
Coppertone Suntan Oil	•					
Sea & Ski Dark Tanning Oil	•					
Sundare Clear Lotion	•					
Swedish Tanning Secret Extra Protection Lotion	•					
Ultima II Highly Protective Tanning Lotion	•					
Aztec Clear Sunscreen Lotion		•				
Block Out		•				
Eclipse		•				
Maxafil		•				
Pabafilm		•				
Pabanol		•				
PreSun		•				
Solbar		•				
SunGard		•				
Uval		•				
A-Fil†			•			
NosKote (for limited body areas)			•			
RVPacque			•			
Zinc Oxide Ointment			•			
QT—Quick Tanning Lotion†				•		
Sea & Ski Indoor/Outdoor Lotion†				•		
Braggi Face Bronzer					•	
Ultima II Ultra Color Gel Stick					•	
Love Spotty Gel—Body Gel					•	
Tanfastic Tanning Butter with Cocoa Butter						•
Tanya Hawaiian Tanning Butter and Coconut Oil						•
Baby Oil (with or without iodine)						•
Mineral Oil (with or without iodine)						•
Lubricating creams and lotions (many brands)						•

*The list of preparations presented in this guide is representative of national brands and does not imply endorsement of any product indicated. No attempt has been made to list every brand of such preparations on the market.
†Also incorporates a chemical sunscreen.

TIPS ON SAFE SUNTANNING

Often a day of sun and fun on the beach is followed by a night of agony and pain from a sunburn. If you are one of the millions who will insist on trying to obtain a "beautiful, healthy tan" this summer, follow these tips to help minimize sunburning:

1. Use your skin coloring as a guide for timing initial sun exposure. Dark-skinned, dark-haired, dark-eyed people generally have more resistance to sunburn than redheads, blonds, and fair-skinned persons.

Generally, those with fair skin should limit their first exposure to no more than 15 to 20 minutes of sun for each side of the body. Increase exposure time by about one-third each day. After a week there should be enough skin thickening and new pigment to provide added protection against burning.

2. Shorten the first exposure in southern latitudes or if you begin exposure in the height of the sunny season.

3. Consider the time of day you will be in the sun. Burning rays are most intense between 11 A.M. and 3 P.M.; sunburn is not likely before 8 A.M. or after 4 P.M.

4. Don't depend on an umbrella to prevent burning. Rays reflected from sand and water can burn even though you are not directly exposed.

5. Don't be fooled by hazy, foggy, or overcast days. These atmospheric conditions scatter the sun's burning rays and may produce a severe sunburn.

6. Observe the tips on suntan preparations given in previous answers in this chapter, and protect yourself against the risk of burning your skin.

21

Other Skin Problems

THE STRUCTURE AND FUNCTION OF SKIN

Can you tell me something about the skin's anatomy and functions? I need this information for a school project.

We are all aware of what the surface of the skin looks like, and we know that it provides many of the physical characteristics that determine an acceptable appearance. But we often fail to think of the skin as a vital, complex organ of the body that performs many important functions.

The skin is one of the largest organs, and receives one-third of all the blood circulating through the body. It varies in thickness from about 1/50 inch on the eyelids to as much as one-third to one-half inch on the upper back. The hair and nails are appendages of the skin, and the sweat glands, oil glands, and mammary glands are accessories of the skin.

The skin of the average adult has over 3,000 square inches of surface area, and fat-free skin accounts for at least 6 percent of an individual's total weight. Thus, the fat-free skin of a 150-pound person weighs at least 9 pounds. One square centimeter contains approximately 15 sebaceous glands, 100 sweat glands, 10 hairs, 1 yard of blood vessels, 4 yards of nerves with 3,000 sensory cells at the ends of nerve fibers, 200 nerve endings to record pain, 25 pressure receptors for the perception of tactile stimuli, 2 sensory receptors for cold, and 12 sensory receptors for heat.

One of the obvious and important functions of the skin is

to protect the rest of the body from the invasion of bacteria and other organisms. It also protects the more sensitive tissues within the body from injury, the sun's rays, the penetration of most harmful chemicals and other agents in the environment, and loss of moisture.

The skin also serves as an organ of perception for the nervous system through its pain, pressure, heat, and cold receptors.

The skin helps to regulate body temperature by constricting blood vessels in response to cold to conserve the body's heat, and by dilating blood vessels and secreting sweat from the sweat glands in response to heat to reduce body temperature. The skin has other functions that we still don't know much about or clearly understand, such as antibody protection.

Like other organs of the body, the skin is subject to abuse, damage, and disease, perhaps even more so because it is visible and unprotected. Because of the skin's visibility and cosmetic importance, however, we seem to be less tolerant and understanding of skin diseases—especially those that are chronic—than we are of diseases affecting other organs.

PRICKLY HEAT

What causes prickly heat and what treatment is advised? Prickly heat (miliaria) is an acute disorder of the sweat mechanism caused by temporary blockage of the sweat duct openings on the skin surface. When sweat cannot reach the skin's surface and a person is subjected to a stimulus—such as heat—that provokes sweating, newly formed sweat may break through the wall of its duct and create an inflammation of the skin. This disorder is manifested as pinhead-sized pimples and blisters, usually accompanied by itching and burning. Heat and moisture may aggravate the condition and allow microorganisms to invade, producing a secondary infection.

Miliaria is especially common in areas where skin surfaces are close together. Thus, it commonly occurs in the skin folds of plump babies and overweight adults.

An important part of treatment is keeping the skin cool and dry. Light, loose-fitting clothes, air conditioning or fans, cool showers followed by the use of dusting powder, and limited physical activity are helpful. Babies with prickly heat should be bathed in plain water, and a physician should be consulted if the prickly heat is severe.

SKIN CARE DURING PREGNANCY

Is any special skin care necessary during pregnancy?
The skin is essentially unaltered in pregnancy. The healthy pregnant woman should therefore continue to carry out her usual cosmetic and skin care procedures.

There are, however, certain internal and skin diseases that tend to be aggravated or initiated by bodily changes that occur during pregnancy. Pigmented moles, freckles, and birthmarks tend to become darker in color, and increased pigmentation (the so-called "mask of pregnancy") may appear on the forehead, cheeks, abdomen, or elsewhere. Little blood vessel enlargements may appear as red spots or as spiderlike tracings anywhere on the skin surface, and streaks may appear on the abdomen or thighs.

These changes, which are within the normal range, need not cause alarm and do not require any special cosmetic attention. However, if isolated brown moles or birthmarks grow rapidly or other unusual skin conditions develop, such as swelling, blistering, or severe, persistent itching, a physician should be consulted at once for diagnosis and necessary treatment.

STRETCH MARKS

I have developed stretch marks from pregnancy. What causes them and can they be removed?
At present there is no way to remove stretch marks (striae). They develop from distension of the skin and are most common when a rapid weight gain is followed by a weight loss, as

in pregnancy. Most pregnant women develop striae; the over-stretched skin is apparently unable to resume its former condition.

An additional factor that may play a role during pregnancy is the increase in certain hormones that promotes the appearance of stretch marks. This has been shown to occur when those hormones are increased during certain disease states, and also when they are administered as medications. Of great importance also is the genetic background of the individual; some people develop stretch marks much more easily than others under similar conditions.

FEVER BLISTERS

I am frequently bothered by fever blisters or cold sores. What causes them and what can I do to prevent them? The common fever blister—or cold sore, as it is often called—results from a virus infection of the skin called herpes simplex. Once the herpes simplex virus infects the skin, it probably resides there in some form, living and reproducing itself without producing skin lesions. At most times the body keeps the virus and its reproduction in check, but certain stimuli can activate or stimulate this virus-producing system in the skin and an eruption results. The eruption consists of a small group of minute blisters filled with a yellowish fluid. Its first indication, usually itching and burning, is followed by tenderness and pain; the blisters dry up and leave a crust that falls off as healing takes place. Scars seldom result except in severe cases.

Colds, menstruation, illness accompanied by fever, trauma such as results from stretching the lip in dental work, and exposure to sun and wind are among the stimuli that can activate the virus-producing system within the skin cells to produce fever blisters.

Since most people have some degree of immunity to the herpes simplex virus, eruptions usually are limited both in the number of people infected and in the severity, area and size of eruption. However, the lesions are not localized to the lip and may occur elsewhere on the skin. In rare cases, when immunity does not exist (especially on first exposure of a young child to the virus), a more extensive outbreak of herpes simplex occurs. Also, in people who are particularly susceptible or lack virus immunity, lesions can recur in the same locations when exposure to the activating agent or event is repeated.

As a rule, fever blisters heal themselves in 2 or 3 weeks or less, with or without treatment. A number of preparations may relieve local discomfort, although it is not certain that they speed healing of the blisters. Observe caution in using popular remedies, since some may cause additional irritation.

A series of smallpox vaccinations and a number of other treatments, including autovaccination (vaccination with the blister fluid), have been used in an attempt to provide immunity from severe recurrent attacks of fever blisters. Their value is not clearly established, although an occasional patient seems to benefit from them.

TREATMENT OF ECZEMA

What causes eczema and what can be done for it?
The word "eczema" has different meanings to different people. It does not refer to a single skin disease; rather it describes a group of skin eruptions characterized by inflammation, redness, swelling, and vesicles. Vesicles are very small blisters formed by the collection of tissue fluids in the upper layers of the skin.

Vesicle formation is quite characteristic of eczema. Large numbers of these tiny blisters are often grouped together. This description would include dermatitis resulting from a reaction to surface contact with compounds to which the patient is allergic (contact dermatitis), but contact dermatitis is usually excluded by definition from the group of skin disorders known as eczema.

Since eczema is often accompanied by itching that causes the patient to scratch the area, the top layers of skin are destroyed and tissue fluid may leak out and become coagulated, forming dry crusts on the skin surface. Rupture of the small vesicles also contributes to crust formation. Repeated scratching may cause the skin to become thickened and rough. Areas of eczema may become secondarily infected by bacteria, with the formation of small abscesses or pustules.

The first step in treatment is establishment of the diagnosis by a physician. Most often the patient comes to the doctor with an eczematous eruption that has been present for a long period of time. It may have been treated with many different local medications that may have modified its appearance. Therefore, the physician must determine how much of the eruption represents the primary process, how much has been caused by locally applied creams or lotions that may have caused irritation of the skin, and what is merely the result of the patient's scratching or digging with fingernails.

Once a proper diagnosis has been made, the physician can prescribe a preparation to reduce the itchiness so that injury to the skin from scratching will be minimized. Other preparations may be prescribed to combat inflammation and infection.

If a physician is not readily available, the golden rule is not to cause further irritation. This is extremely important, since the inflamed skin has lost its normal protective power. Wet compresses of lukewarm water can be applied to the affected area two or three times a day. A bland ointment can also be applied until a physician can be consulted.

TREATMENT OF KERATOSES

What causes keratoses? Are they dangerous and can they be removed?

A keratosis is one type of localized overgrowth involving the horny (outer) layer of the skin. (Other conditions such as calluses are also an overgrowth of the horny layer.) Of several types of keratoses, seborrheic and actinic are the most common.

It is important to distinguish between these forms, since seborrheic keratoses do not become malignant while actinic keratoses are premalignant; a small percentage will become malignant if untreated.

Seborrheic keratoses occur primarily on the trunk of the body, though they can appear on the face and scalp. They vary greatly in appearance and size: some contain little pigment; others are jet black in color; all are raised above the skin surface. With age these lesions tend to increase in size and number; some people have hundreds. Seborrheic keratoses do not require treatment unless they are being irritated or are a cosmetic problem.

Actinic keratoses, in contrast, consist of growths of cells into the skin and are much harder to describe in simple terms. Usually they appear as red, scaly areas of various sizes, primarily on exposed areas of the body (face, arms and hands), and are more common in people with a history of heavy sun exposure. Actinic keratoses should be treated to prevent possible malignancy. A physician can treat and eliminate keratoses in many ways and without much difficulty.

PSORIASIS

My husband has been troubled with psoriasis for 10 years. His nails are completely deformed and his psoriasis has spread, in patches, to about 40 percent of his body. What causes this condition? What treatments are available?

Psoriasis (pronounced so-rye-ah-sis) is a skin disorder that affects at least one out of fifty people in the United States. It is characterized by thickened, reddened, silver-scaled patches of skin that may appear as a few small lesions or cover large areas of the body. When the nails are involved, you may notice a loss of luster, small pits or cross-ridgings on nail surfaces, and loosening of the nail from its bed.

Since other skin conditions may resemble psoriasis, anyone who thinks he or she has psoriasis should consult a physician for diagnosis and treatment.

Although researchers have not discovered the exact cause of psoriasis or its cure, much is known about this disease. What once was considered a hopeless, incurable condition can now be controlled when therapeutic measures are conscientiously applied.

The extent of discomfort from psoriasis is a factor in determining treatment. A physician may prescribe various ointments, creams, lotions, and/or several forms of internal therapy.

PSORIASIS CAN BE HELPED

What is the current status of treatment for psoriasis?
There is no specific treatment for psoriasis. The patient should allow a physician who has considerable experience with measures that may be effective to treat the problem. Although there is no known cure, medications and other treatments may reduce or control the skin rash. Therapy, properly prescribed and followed, can in a limited number of patients clear the disease completely for many years. In other cases, benefits may be partial or last for a shorter time.

More often than not, therapy must be used intermittently, or even continuously, to keep the disease under control. Psoriasis tends to clear up spontaneously, often for long periods of time, so that it is difficult to assess the value of remedies used.

There is no reason for the patient with psoriasis to avoid treatment and just "learn to live with the disease." Some form of beneficial therapy may reduce suffering and disfigurement, even if it does not cure.

NO NEW CURE FOR PSORIASIS

*I have suffered from psoriasis for 20 years. Now a friend
tells me that there is a simple, inexpensive, and rapid cure
for it. Is this true?*

Your friend is incorrect. There still is no cure for psoriasis.
Your friend probably read an ad for one of the numerous
products promoted for psoriasis. (Sometimes these ads are
written like regular news articles to make the reader think a
breakthrough has been made.) The cause of psoriasis is still
unknown, despite much research, and there is no treatment
that is best for all patients. Most of the products used to treat
psoriasis contain coal-tar derivatives combined with other ingredients to help remove the scales that characterize the condition. Some people are helped by these products. But since
psoriasis has a tendency to flare up and then subside, and since
it may be either mild and localized or severe and widespread,
no one product or therapeutic approach will benefit everyone.
A physician can select the treatment that may be most effective for a specific person.

Treatments include various ointments, creams, lotions,
several forms of internal therapy, and physical therapy such
as carefully regulated exposure to ultraviolet light (of a specific
wavelength only) or sunlight. Some present-day treatments do
appear promising, but it is still too early for a final evaluation.

Psoriasis is a chronic disease (like arthritis or diabetes).
It can be controlled, but it cannot be cured. Most patients can
be helped by treatment, but control entails periodic visits to
the doctor and careful adherence to the treatment prescribed.
Too often, when the condition begins to improve or temporarily clears, the patient stops using medication and stops
visiting a physician. Then the psoriasis flares up again and the
patient is distraught. Understanding and cooperation on the
part of the patient are the most important aspects of successful
treatment of this disease.

RINGWORM

Our son has ringworm of the scalp and we are wondering where he caught it. What causes ringworm? What is the best treatment?

"Ringworm" is the popular name for superficial fungal infections of the skin. The name is apparently derived from the appearance of the skin lesions, which are often round and spread from the center outward in circles or rings. Fungal infections of the scalp often appear in this type of pattern with one or more gray patches covered with yellow scales and dry, fragile hairs. The affected hairs may break off close to the scalp, producing a bald appearance.

Fungal infections of the scalp are most often seen in children and are contagious. Several different species of fungus may be responsible for infections. The fungus may be picked up from close contact with an infected person, dog, or cat. Barber clippers, combs, and hats may also be sources of infection.

It is best to consult a physician for proper diagnosis and treatment of such fungal infections. Various medications may be applied to the scalp to treat the infection topically, but physicians most often prescribe a drug, griseofulvin. This drug is taken internally and provides clearing within a short period of time for most cases of ringworm. The hair should be shampooed daily and in most cases any shampoo will do, although physicians may sometimes prescribe special shampoos. The physician may remove weakened, infected hairs from the involved areas with adhesive tape and may recommend clipping the hairs close to the scalp. Removal of the infected hairs reduces the spread of infection. The scalp need not be shaved, as was done in the past.

In most instances children can still attend school regularly, since griseofulvin prevents spreading of the fungal spores and minimizes the risk of disseminating the infection. It is not advisable for the child to be required to wear a cap, since children tend to trade headgear, which promotes rather than prevents spread of the infection.

WARTS: CAUSE AND TREATMENT

What causes warts? Are there different kinds of warts?
A wart results from a viral infection of the epidermis, the outer layer of skin. Warts also can be described as virus-caused growths. Since today it is believed that most warts are caused by the same virus, they are classified by location; this is not only easier, but makes more sense because problems are related to location rather than cause. For example, plantar warts derive their name from the plantar surface (soles) of the feet, where they occur, often causing a great deal of discomfort. Warts can develop on any part of the skin, but appear most often on the hands, fingers, and soles, apparently because these areas come into contact with the virus most frequently. Warts are contagious and the virus can be transmitted from one person to another.

Most people are susceptible to the virus, and almost all of us develop warts at some time in our lives. Adults are less likely to have warts than children, possibly because of an acquired immunization—a buildup of antibodies—that develops as a person grows older. Apparently a person can be totally immune or resistant to warts, since despite contact with the virus, some people never get them.

Most warts eventually disappear without treatment. A person who wants a wart removed should consult a physician who can offer several methods of treatment. Remedies for warts that can be bought without a prescription usually contain some kind of acid and can be harmful if the directions are not followed carefully.

WITCHING WARTS AWAY

Is it true that warts can be "charmed" away?
If a wart sufferer believes in a certain treatment—no matter how ridiculous or unscientific—that treatment sometimes seems to cure the warts. Folk "cures" such as rubbing warts with grasshopper's "tobacco spit," milkweed juice, or ear wax and tales of "witching" warts away are hundreds of years old. Mark Twain recorded several methods of curing warts in *The Adventures of Tom Sawyer*—among them, burying a cat at midnight where some wicked person lies buried.

A logical explanation for such "cures" is that warts can disappear spontaneously. But if the disappearance of the wart and use of the "cure" happen to coincide in time, no amount of logic will prevail with some "folk medicine" believers.

PLANTAR WARTS

How do plantar warts differ from other warts?
Plantar warts occur on the soles (plantar surfaces) of the feet. Because trauma plays an important part in the development of warts, plantar warts occur most often on points of pressure. They are generally considered one of the most serious and troublesome types of warts because they can be very painful, and even disabling. Unlike warts on other body areas, plantar warts are flattened and pushed inward and sideways by the pressure of walking. This may squeeze nerve endings, causing pain.

It is always wise to consult a physician concerning plantar warts. Cooperation with the physician is important, and a patient should not demand removal of these warts, since in some cases such treatment may produce scarring that is permanent and may be as painful as the warts.

REDNESS OF THE FACE

My doctor tells me I have rosacea. What causes this condition and what is the recommended treatment?

Rosacea is a disease characterized by redness of the central area of the face due to dilation (which can be fleeting or lasting) of small blood vessels, often accompanied by an oily skin and the appearance of acnelike pimples in the same areas. Conjuctiva and corneas may also be involved.

The cause of this condition is totally unknown. Recent studies suggest that some changes in the lining of the stomach and intestines accompany rosacea, but it is difficult to tell whether this is the cause of the disease or an associated disturbance. The results of earlier studies were conflicting.

When rosacea does appear, it is often aggravated by emotional factors, by exposure to hot and cold weather and wind, by ingestion of alcoholic or spicy beverages and foods, and by irritants in general.

The treatment of rosacea depends on the stage and severity of the disease, age of the patient, and other factors. Calming agents and antibiotics may be taken internally. Drying and antiseptic, as well as soothing, local preparations may be prescribed. Elimination of some of the redness may be accomplished by electrolysis or desiccation. The type of treatment should be decided by a dermatologist, and may have to be changed according to the patient's response. The aggravating factors mentioned earlier should be avoided.

RHINOPHYMA

My nose has become large and misshapen on the end, with small dilated blood vessels. Everyone kids me and says it is caused by drinking too much, even though I don't overindulge. What is the real cause of this condition? What treatment is recommended?

The scientific name for the condition in which the nose becomes red and misshapen on the end is rhinophyma.

It is a severe form of rosacea (see previous exchange) in which there is a thickened, lobulated overgrowth of skin and connective tissue and sebaceous glands with dilated blood vessels on the lower half of the nose. Other midline facial areas may be similarly involved. The condition primarily affects middle-aged and older men; it is almost nonexistent in women. The overgrowth of the nose may at times be quite large and presents a severe cosmetic and social defect.

The exact cause of rhinophyma is not known, and many things have been reported as possible causative or aggravating factors. Overindulgence in tea, coffee, alcohol, and spiced or very hot foods and drinks is widely accepted as a cause, although the condition may occur in people who never drink or smoke. Others think rhinophyma is associated with digestive disorders, or with a parasite that invades the skin's follicles. Psychological factors have been emphasized by some; tension, excitement, or fatigue unquestionably heighten the flushing in some patients.

The condition is chronic but is treatable. Every effort should be made to avoid those factors that cause flushing or dilation of capillaries. Exposure to extremes of heat and cold should be minimized. Hot drinks, coffee, tea, spices, and alcohol should be completely avoided for a test period of at least one month, although it is found that in some patients any or all of these may be ingested without any effect on the redness. Anything that relieves tension is desirable; emotional disturbances should be avoided as much as possible.

Various topical and internal medications may also be helpful in the early stages of rhinophyma. Large, broken blood vessels may be destroyed by electrolysis or superficial electrodesiccation. In advanced stages, the best treatment for rhinophyma is surgery. Under local, or sometimes general, anesthesia, the nose can be reshaped by the removal of superfluous tissue. This is done with a scalpel, a dermoplaning instrument, an electrosurgical unit, or a combination of these techniques.

LUMPS IN THE ARMPIT

Periodically I get a small, hard lump under my arm. What causes this and what treatment is recommended?

Lumps in the armpit can have several causes. They may be caused by an allergic reaction to one particular ingredient found in some antiperspirants. However, this reaction is probably less common than it was a few years ago because most offending agents have been removed from antiperspirants now available.

Another cause of a lump in the armpit can be a boil. Usually the bacteria that produce the boil enter through a hair follicle; however, the armpits contain specialized sweat glands, and some boils involve these glands. When this occurs, the lesions become more difficult to manage and tend to be chronic. Surgery may be necessary.

A third cause of a lump may be a cyst. (See the next question on cysts and boils.)

Finally, the lump may represent enlargement of one or more lymph glands, more properly called lymph nodes. The most common cause of such an enlargement is an infection of the lower arm or hand. However, the nodes may become enlarged as a result of many other conditions, some of which are serious and require immediate treatment.

Since the causes of a lump in the armpit are so varied, it would be wise to consult a physician for diagnosis and treatment if you notice such swelling.

CYSTS AND BOILS

What is the difference between a cyst and a boil?

These two lesions are entirely different. A boil is an abscess of the skin caused by an infection with pus-forming bacteria. Boils usually form in infected hair follicles. The lesion is a tender, hot, red mass and can be very sore. There may be a small central white area or a draining area. The material that drains from the boil is a mixture of germs, cells, and tissues that have been destroyed in the inflammatory reaction.

In contrast, a cyst is a noninflamed, saclike structure completely lined with a layer of skinlike material. Usually it is neither tender nor hot. Cysts may begin as plugged glands of one kind or another, or may result from pieces of skin being buried beneath the surface. There may be a small opening in the cyst through which the contents drain. In contrast to the material in a boil, this material consists of the products of the cells that form the cyst wall. Sometimes a cyst ruptures or becomes infected and inflamed and has the same clinical appearance as a boil.

TREATMENT OF BOILS

What causes boils and what treatment is recommended? Boils are infections of the skin usually caused by a type of bacteria known as staphylococci. Clinically, they are manifested as large, tender, warm, raised, red areas that may involve a small central yellow area of pus.

Since boils are true infections of the skin that may appear as acnelike lesions, particularly in the scalp and underarm areas, consultation with a physician is needed. Especially in patients with recurrent boils, the physician must not rule out the possibility of an underlying disease, such as diabetes, in which there is a predisposition for the development of boils.

Depending on the nature of the lesion, the physician may incise the boil to promote drainage. Of course the lesions may drain by themselves. The patient must avoid squeezing the boil, since squeezing may spread the infection.

Treatment of acute conditions should include the use of hot compresses for 10 to 15 minutes at least four times a day. The physician may use antibiotics as well as other medications in treatment.

An important part of therapy is preventing the appearance of new lesions. The patient is advised to take a shower with soap or detergent incorporating an antiseptic twice a day. When lesions recur frequently, underclothing and bed linen should be changed every day.

ITCH FROM GLASS FIBERS

Why does material made from glass fibers cause the skin to itch? How can washing curtains of this type in a washing machine with other clothes cause an itching skin rash? Itching from contact with these fabrics is due to irritation of the skin by tiny, needlelike particles of the glass fibers. Several cases of itchy skin eruptions have been traced to washing glass-fiber curtains in a washing machine along with the family underwear or just prior to washing the family clothes. Evidently, the tiny particles of glass fibers become attached to the clothes and cause skin irritation when the clothes are worn.

Since today's curtains, bedspreads and other items are often made of these fabrics, everyone should be alert to the possible development of skin irritations if these fabrics come in contact with clothes through washing. In the past, some manufacturers' laundering directions stated that their glass-fiber fabrics could be washed in machines, but the Federal Government has passed a regulation prohibiting such statements and requiring that a warning be included with glass-fiber fabrics stating that skin irritation may occur if they are washed in machines. Read the label accompanying glass-fiber fabrics, and wash them by hand following the manufacturer's directions.

SKIN REACTIONS TO SPANDEX

Is it true that foundation garments containing spandex may cause allergic skin reactions? Several doctors have reported allergic skin reactions caused by the synthetic elastic fiber known as spandex.

Since spandex washes and wears better than rubber, it is replacing rubber in many stretch fabrics. In the United States, spandex fibers are sold under the following trademarks: Lycra, Glospan, Spandelle, Duraspan, and Vyrene. A variety of women's garments, including swimsuits, foundation garments, stretch pants, and stockings now contain spandex, and it is also being used in men's clothing—elastic tops of socks and waistbands of pants and underwear.

If you develop a skin reaction such as redness or itching in areas that come in contact with a spandex garment, you may be allergic to spandex and should avoid it in the future. The clothing label will indicate whether it contains spandex. If the skin reaction is uncomfortable or doesn't clear quickly, see a physician for treatment.

SKIN REACTIONS FROM TIGHT PANTS

My mother says I should stop wearing tight-fitting pants because they cause itchy skin rashes on thighs and legs. Is this true? All of my friends wear pants like these, and I don't want to stop unless it's really dangerous.

Some physicians have noted an increased number of skin reactions among adolescent and young adult males who wear trousers with an extremely narrow cut to the legs. These include red, itchy, and scaling dermatitis of the scrotum, inflamed hair follicles on the front surfaces of the thighs, exaggeration of "winter itch," and other skin reactions on the thighs and legs.

Reactions appear in two forms: (1) a nondescript red, itchy, slightly scaling skin eruption confined to the body area covered by the tight pants, and perhaps most severe where the pants bind most closely; or (2) an exaggeration, in areas covered by the tight pants, of already existing skin problems.

These skin eruptions are produced by mechanical pressure or friction; they are not allergic reactions. Such factors as movement of the skin surface under the pants as the body moves, and the tropical environment of the skin—increased heat and humidity caused by the tight fit—are aggravating factors.

These reactions have been called "stretch-garment dermatitis" because physicians first saw them in girls whose acne on the shoulders and back was aggravated by wearing tight-fitting stretch bras.

If you develop any skin reaction such as those described above, stop wearing tight pants and consult your physician for treatment.

HEADBAND DERMATITIS

I like to wear headbands to hold my long hair off my face, but my forehead has broken out in a rash. Could the headband be the cause?

Indeed it could. Leather headbands may produce an allergic skin reaction that resembles the classic "hatband dermatitis" seen in some men who wear hats with leather bands. The wearer is allergic to one of the tanning chemicals or dyes used on the leather.

Another type of skin reaction produced by headbands is an eruption resembling acne that may appear underneath various kinds of headbands. This reaction is most likely due to increased sweating, irritating mechanical factors, or acne-producing resins acting on the skin of people in the acne-susceptible age group.

A third type of skin reaction is caused by various headband ornamentations that contain or are composed of substances such as essential oils, lacquers, plastics, or dyes. These reactions may be allergic in nature, or the substance may be a "primary irritant" (a substance that acts as an irritant to the skin of most people who come in contact with it).

Armbands and necklaces may produce the same kinds of reactions as headbands.

If a skin reaction develops underneath a headband, armband, or necklace, stop wearing it. If the reaction disappears when the band is no longer worn, the band is probably the cause. It may be possible to wear bands made of different materials (leather instead of beaded or vice versa) unless the reaction is of the acne type, in which case the only recourse is to stop wearing headbands or to wear them for only short periods of time. It may be necessary to consult a physician if the skin reaction does not disappear.

SKIN REACTIONS TO HANDMADE JEWELRY

I have some handmade jewelry that I like very much, but every time I wear it I break out in a rash. The jewelry looks like silver, but I'm not sure it is. Is there anything I can do that would allow me to wear it?

Jewelry that contains nickel alloy often causes allergic skin reactions. If you buy an item that is not marked sterling silver or 14-karat (or heavier) gold, it is likely to contain nickel. The metal used for handcrafted or costume jewelry, watchbands, and the backs of wristwatches very frequently contains nickel alloy.

You might try coating the part of your jewelry that touches your skin with a layer of clear fingernail polish. If this does not keep you from developing the rash, you will have to stop wearing the jewelry.

ALLERGY TO LEATHER

I recently purchased a pair of leather sandals made in India, but I wore them a few times and developed a rash on my feet. Why would these sandals cause a skin reaction when none of my other leather sandals do? Can I do anything to prevent the rash?

The reactions are caused by an allergic sensitivity to ingredients used in the tanning process. In Europe and in the United States, leather is usually tanned with chromates (chemicals), but Indian leather is often cured with vegetable tannins, some of which are similar to poison ivy plants.

It is believed that these vegetable tannins are responsible for allergic reactions to leather sandals from India.

If you have reacted to your Indian leather sandals, your only recourse is to stop wearing them. If the skin reaction does not disappear, consult a physician.

LANOLIN AND WOOL SENSITIVITY

I cannot wear woolen garments without itching and breaking out in a rash. Should I also avoid products that contain lanolin?

Although people who are allergic to wool have commonly been warned that they may also be allergic to lanolin, there is serious doubt that the two allergies go hand in hand.

About the only thing lanolin and wool have in common is that they are both derived from sheep, lanolin being analogous to sebum (natural oil on the skin) and wool to hair. Their chemical compositions and antigenic compounds are entirely different and do not cross-react. It is doubtful that any lanolin present on sheep hair at the time of shearing remains on wool fibers through processing. The fibers are thoroughly cleaned and scoured in the manufacturing of yarn, fabrics, and finally clothes. Of course, you could be allergic to both wool and lanolin, but these would be two separate allergies.

CAUSE OF CHAPPED SKIN

What causes chapping of the skin?

The skin's outer layer is highly flexible. This flexibility depends on proper hydration of keratin, the protein substance that makes up this layer. Dehydration causes loss of flexibility and considerable brittleness, which leads to cracks—the condition commonly referred to as chapped skin.

This problem usually occurs when there is a sudden drop in humidity, as in cold weather, because in a cold, dry atmosphere the skin's outer layer loses water to the air. Frequent contact with water, incomplete drying of the skin, and excessive use of soaps, detergents, and other chemicals may reduce the outer layer's water-holding capacity so that chapping results. Inflammation of the skin may follow chapping if these conditions are not corrected promptly.

TREATMENT OF CHAPPED SKIN

Every year I suffer from dry, chapped skin. What can I do about it?

To avoid dry, chapped skin, avoid the things that cause chapping. Don't overdo it with soap when bathing. Use warm (not hot) water for showers and baths. Adding a capful of bath oil to the tub will help too. While your skin is still wet, apply a thin film of bland, unmedicated cream or lotion and then towel dry. The cream will help retard evaporation of moisture from your skin. Keep your home adequately humidified during the dry winter months. Apply creams and lotions frequently to your hands and face, and always dry your hands thoroughly after they have been in water.

BAGS UNDER THE EYES

What causes "bags" under eyes?

Changes in the skin under the eyes that lead to pouching, commonly called "bags," are primarily due to heredity and usually occur with advancing age. Normally the skin of the eyelids is delicate and loosely attached. As a person grows older, some underlying muscles and tissues are lost, and the lower lids tend to fall in folds. Underlying fat pushes through weakened muscles, causing the baggy tissue to balloon out.

If extreme, this may constitute a disfigurement that is a social and economic handicap, especially when it occurs in a young person. Cosmetics offer little or no help. Plastic surgery is the only method that will improve this condition. For details, see Chapter 22, "Esthetic Surgery."

This permanent skin change is considerably different from the puffy eyelids that may signal the presence of severe kidney or heart disease. Mild recurring allergies and chronic skin disorders may also cause puffiness because this area with its loosely attached skin is particularly apt to accumulate fluid.

In elderly persons with impaired circulation, puffiness of upper and lower lids may be obvious at the end of the day due to fluid accumulation. Or fluid may accumulate in the eyelid on the side of the face that is down during sleep. Improvement in these conditions depends on discovering and correcting underlying causes.

DARK CIRCLES UNDER EYES

What causes dark circles under eyes? Do they indicate that anything is wrong physically?

Dark circles under the eyes usually have no relation to physical disease; the condition depends on several anatomic factors and may reflect a family trait. The skin of the eyelids is thin and contains little fatty tissue. Blood that passes through large veins close to the surface shows through the skin, producing a bluish-black tint.

Darkening circles are accentuated when one is tired and pale, during menstruation, and in the latter part of pregnancy. With aging, the discoloration may become more obvious and permanent.

Special cosmetics, usually modifications of makeup bases, are available at the cosmetic counters of most large drug and department stores to cover dark circles. Those who wear glasses may find that tinted lenses will help make dark circles under their eyes less noticeable.

BROKEN BLOOD VESSELS ON LEGS

I have broken blood vessels on my legs, which I find unattractive. What can I do to conceal or get rid of them?

Broken veins or capillaries are popular terms for the bluish-red discolorations that occur on the legs, often in the shape of a spider web. These blemishes consist of tiny dilated veins filled or congested with blood. They may appear as early as age thirty in areas of greatest strain—on the outer surface of the mid-thighs, just below the knees, and around the ankles.

When these blemishes are accompanied by varicose veins, there may be considerable discomfort. Otherwise, they are significant only because they are so close to the skin's surface that they are cosmetically detracting. The color is often so intense that they look like bruises; this is particularly disturbing when bathing suits are worn. Several brands of special leg makeup designed to tone down the deep purple-red discoloration are available, but they will not completely mask the blemishes.

Some people believe that any practice or activity that makes it difficult for blood to circulate freely should be avoided. This includes restrictions such as circular garters, tight girdles, keeping legs crossed while sitting, prolonged standing, and excessive walking. In some instances, moderate muscular exercise, such as walking, is useful.

A physician should be consulted if there is any discomfort or concern, or if broken blood vessels occur on the trunk of the body or on the face. While such blemishes resemble the dilated veins discussed above, they may be associated with other disorders.

ENLARGED BLOOD VESSELS ON THE FACE

I am forty years old. Recently small blood vessels have begun to show on my nose and have spread over my face. Is there any way to prevent this? Is there a method to remove, conceal, or reduce the redness of those already present?

From your description, the enlarged blood vessels appear to be the type classified as telangiectases. Such changes have many possible causes including heredity, excessive exposure to sunlight, liver damage, and a skin disease known as rosacea. Examination by a physician would be necessary to differentiate among these causes.

Further telangiectasia can be prevented in some instances, depending on the cause of the condition. Exposure to cold, wind, sun, and heat, rapid changes in temperature, and very hot or highly spiced foods and beverages should, generally, be avoided.

The cosmetic defect can be minimized by appropriate makeup. Choice of treatment, if required, is best left to the examining physician, who has available all of the facts in your case. Electrodesiccation (destruction of the lesions by careful use of an electric needle) and cryosurgery (freezing with dry ice [carbon dioxide snow] or liquid nitrogen) are among the treatments that may be recommended. Such treatments are safe and effective when performed by a physician.

ALLERGY TO BEE STINGS

I am allergic to bee stings. What do you recommend in terms of prevention and treatment?

Since severe reactions and even death may occur in persons allergic to bee stings, you should consult a physician who will supply you with medication to carry for emergency use if you are stung by a bee. Your physician may also try immunization (hyposensitization), particularly if you are exposed to bees frequently; however, hyposensitization has not been perfected and is not always effective.

You can protect yourself in several ways. Wear white or light-colored clothes instead of dark colors, since light colors do not attract or antagonize bees. Avoid using perfumes, hair spray, hair tonic, suntan lotions, and similar cosmetics—bees are attracted to their odor—and always wear shoes outdoors. People who have severe allergies to bee stings can also wear protective nets when they are near bees or run the risk of being stung.

If you are stung by a honeybee, try to remove the stinger and attached venom sac as soon as possible without applying pressure to the sac. Hornets, wasps, and yellow jackets, which do not leave their stingers, should be brushed off quickly. For immediate relief from a sting, apply ice or cold compresses to the area. Avoid strong agents and any treatment that may further irritate your skin, and remember that the practice of applying mud to bee and wasp stings can lead to infection. If the swelling increases or you notice any difficulty in breathing, see a doctor at once.

CHIGGER BITES

I plan to go camping this month. What kind of repellents or other methods of protection will help prevent chigger bites?

Chiggers are the larvae of various mites. They are common in the southern United States during summer months and are found in bushes, fields, and moist, swampy places.

Naturally, the best protection is to avoid chigger habitats. However, this is almost impossible when camping and hiking in wooded areas. In such circumstances, treating your clothing with repellents provides protection from chiggers (as well as from ticks and fleas). If your clothing does not cover vulnerable skin areas, treat your skin also.

No repellent as yet is completely satisfactory, but the more effective ones include diethyltoluamide (deet), dimethyl carbate, and benzyl benzoate. Powdered sulfur has also been used. Check the label to determine whether the product you plan to purchase contains one of these chemicals as an active ingredient.

The simplest way to treat clothing is to shake about a dozen drops of the repellent into one palm, rub your hands together, and rub the repellent lightly on socks, shirts, blouses, or slacks where bites tend to occur. Apply liberally along all openings of your clothing (insides of neckbands, cuffs of trousers, and tops of socks), repeating until you have covered all areas to be treated. If you are using a spray-type product, simply spray the same areas. All repellents except benzyl benzoate are removed by washing.

To protect your skin, shake a few drops from the bottle or spray from the pressurized can into your palms, smear evenly, then apply thoroughly to the backs of your hands, wrists, neck, ears, face, and any other exposed skin. Use enough repellent to provide a uniform film.

Despite these precautions, you still may be bitten by chiggers. If so, bathe as soon as the chigger bites are noticed to help remove them from your skin. Cooling lotions such as calamine may help relieve itching and irritation.

If you are very uncomfortable, a physician will be able to prescribe appropriate additional medication.

PANTY HOSE VAGINITIS

Is it true that wearing panty hose can cause vaginal infections?

Panty hose themselves cannot cause vaginal infections. However, they do provide a warm, moist environment where the organisms that cause vaginal infections can grow. This in turn can cause symptoms of unusual vaginal inflammation such as discharges and vulval itching. If you are bothered by vaginal infections but don't have any internal problems and don't use local birth control devices or feminine deodorant products, any tight-fitting garments—including panty hose—are suspect.

POISON IVY

I'm fond of the outdoors but seem to be a magnet for poison ivy. What treatment is recommended for it, and

*can I be immunized against it? Can I wash the affected
areas and wear loose clothing to hide the blisters?*

The only satisfactory way to prevent poison ivy rash is to avoid
the plants that cause it. There is as yet no skin protectant or
immunizing technique generally available. Poison ivy plants
contain compounds (catechols) that produce redness and
blisters (dermatitis). Erroneously called poisons, the compounds are allergens—substances that can cause a person to
react unfavorably when exposed to them.

If you think you have been exposed to poison ivy, wash
your skin with soap and water as soon as possible to help reduce the chances of developing a dermatitis. Soap helps to
remove the allergen. Your hands especially should be washed
because, if contaminated, they can spread the dermatitis to
other parts of your body. Also wash clothes, garden imple-
ments, bikes, baseball gloves, or anything else that may have
come in contact with the plant. Once the allergen is removed
by washing, however, there is no further benefit from washing
and scrubbing.

The simplest, most practical way to obtain relief from itching and to reduce inflammation is to apply cold-water compresses to the affected areas. Bathing, showering, and other
exposure to water are useful, and even essential, in treatment.
Calamine lotion applied early will hasten the drying of small
blisters.

To treat areas where it is impractical to use wet compresses, take lukewarm baths with water softener added.

Physicians treat extensive eruptions with oral or topical
cortisone remedies; superimposed infections are treated with
antibiotics. Oral antihistaminic drugs can often relieve the
itching. However, local remedies may cause additional inflammation and blistering if the patient is or becomes allergic
to one or more of the ingredients, so it is best to avoid such
products.

Loose clothing can be worn without fear of aggravating

the condition. Contrary to popular belief, breaking the blisters does not cause the dermatitis to "spread."

EXERCISES AND CREAMS FOR A BIGGER BUST

Are there any safe exercises or bust developers that will really increase the size of my breasts? I feel unfeminine with small breasts and can't afford plastic surgery.

The only way you can actually increase the size of your breasts is through plastic surgery. The next best thing is a padded bra —this can at least give the appearance of a bigger bust and may make your clothes fit better. But don't waste your time or money on bust-developing exercises, creams, or devices. None of them work, and some can be dangerous.

Breasts do not contain muscular tissue that can be developed by exercises. But exercise can help improve your posture and develop the pectoral muscles under your breasts—giving the appearance of more fullness. Massaging devices have no redeeming qualities. They can injure breast tissue or spread undetected cancer within the breast. Breast development creams also can be dangerous. Some contain hormones that, if absorbed into the body, can upset the body's own hormone balance. This can disrupt menstrual cycles and may prove harmful to women with unsuspected breast tumors. Your best bet is to stop worrying about the size of your breasts.

Large breasts are not a prerequisite for femininity, satisfactory sexual relations, or breast-feeding. And, since going braless is now considered fashionable by some, small breasts can actually be an asset.

HORMONES TO ENLARGE BREASTS

Please help me with my problem. I want to have a large bustline. I have been told that certain hormones will help enlarge my breasts and that galactagogues like belladonna or atropine are useful for the same purpose. Please tell me how to go about using these hormones.

Belladonna and atropine, the drugs you mention, are neither hormones nor galactagogues and do not increase breast size. Galactagogues are agents that induce or increase secretion of milk from the breasts. Belladonna and atropine do not significantly affect secretion of milk from the breasts and should not be used unless prescribed by a physician.

Preparations and devices that claim to enlarge breasts fall into the category of quackery. They will not increase breast size to any significant degree, and in some cases can actually be harmful. Some of these so-called "bust enlargers" may contain hormones.

Female hormones taken internally may produce a slight breast enlargement during administration, but the breasts return to their original size once the drugs are stopped. This phenomenon has been observed by many women taking oral contraceptives. Physicians usually do not prescribe hormones just to enlarge the breasts, because such hormones are known to produce other changes in the body.

Plastic surgery is the only procedure that will increase breast size to the degree that women concerned about the problem desire. The operation is referred to as breast augmentation. If you are interested in this procedure, consult a physician experienced in plastic surgery. (See Chapter 22, "Esthetic Surgery," for details about breast augmentation.)

DERMOGRAPHISM—"SKIN WRITING"

What causes dermographism, or "skin writing," and is there a cure?
Dermographism is a condition characterized by an exaggerated skin response to minimal injury. Wheals or welts (raised, red marks) appear on skin areas to which normal pressure is applied. Scratching, stroking, or pressure from clothes—especially tight, binding clothes such as bra straps, girdles, belts, or waistbands—will induce whealing and welting. Because the

wheals cause itching, dermographism can be very uncomfortable.

The term "skin writing" has been applied to this condition because stroking or applying pressure firmly on the skin with a fingernail or a bluntly pointed object produces raised, red streaks in the writing pattern.

The cause of dermographism is unknown. It is believed to be allergic in nature and often occurs following other allergic reactions. But it also occurs independently, in otherwise normal people, and without apparent cause.

Dermographism is chronic, can persist for a long time and often disappears gradually, over a period of months or years. The condition is harmless but annoying. There is no cure, but prescription medications can relieve itching and suppress welts.

ICHTHYOSIS—FISH-SCALE SKIN

I have a skin condition called ichthyosis and would appreciate information on its cause and treatment.

Ichthyosis is a fairly common hereditary skin condition characterized by dry scaling and thickening of the skin that resembles fish scales—thus the common name, "fish-scale disease." Severity of the condition ranges from mild to severe, but the milder forms are more common.

Ichthyosis usually becomes evident shortly after birth. It may become somewhat less marked at puberty, when the activity of the oil glands increases greatly, and it is often accentuated with aging, when the skin normally becomes drier and more scaly.

There is no cure for ichthyosis. However, various treatments can greatly improve the appearance of the skin and relieve the excessive dryness and scaling. If you are not under a dermatologist's care, we suggest that you consult one.

GRAPEFRUIT TO BLEACH THE SKIN

I tried to soften and bleach the rough, darkened skin on my elbows by rubbing it with grapefruit halves, but it didn't work. Can you suggest a good commercial bleaching cream or another way to bleach my elbows?

Citrus fruits such as grapefruit and lemons contain mild acids that may have slight bleaching action; however, as you discovered, this action is not sufficient to produce significant bleaching of skin. For better results, you might try one of the bleaching creams made with hydroquinone. They work for many people, although their effectiveness depends on the type of hyperpigmentation. These products may also cause an allergic skin rash in some people, so they should be tried with caution.

If your rough, darkened skin is the result of dryness or chapping, any body cream or lotion will help. You can also try scrubbing your elbows with a brush and soap or gently rubbing them with a pumice stone after bathing. The rubbing action eliminates some of the outer layers of dead, rough skin; but too vigorous rubbing may irritate the areas and increase the problem. If you're especially conscious of the spots, cover them up with a special masking cosmetic.

Sometimes problems such as you describe are caused by medical conditions such as ichthyosis, inverse eczema, thyroid dysfunction, and keratinizing problems. In any case that doesn't respond to the cosmetic procedures mentioned above, it's best to consult your doctor.

CIGARETTE STAINS ON FINGERS

I know it's not healthy for me to smoke cigarettes, but I do it anyway. Will you please tell me how I can get cigarette stains off my fingers and the smell of cigarettes out of my hair?

Perfume, cologne or perfumed hair spray may help to camouflage the smell of cigarettes in your hair, but the only effective way to remove the odor is to wash your hair.

Filtered cigarettes do not seem to stain the skin as much as unfiltered ones do because their tobacco usually doesn't come in contact with one's fingers.

Scrubbing your stained fingers with a brush and soap may help to remove the stain by washing away some of the outer layers of dead skin.

Some people believe that home remedies such as vinegar or lemon juice will bleach out the stain. These products contain acid, which may have a slight bleaching effect, but it is doubtful that this is strong enough to remove any stain.

If you were to stop smoking, it would take about two weeks for the stained cells to be replaced by new, unstained ones.

MAINTAINING "PERFECT" SKIN

What can I do to have a perfect complexion? I take very good care of my skin, but when I look at it closely with a magnifying mirror, I see all kinds of blemishes and bumps. We advise you to throw away your magnifying mirror and stop worrying about your complexion. There is probably no one with such perfect skin that it will not show flaws upon magnification. Certainly other people will not notice blemishes that require magnification to see. The primary skin concern of most people is how it looks to others. Others rarely get close enough to note variations in your skin texture.

If you are preoccupied with the appearance of your skin, you will not only create problems where they don't exist or are minimal, but you will succeed in drawing the attention of others to your concern.

"ACID MANTLE"

*I have seen references to the "acid mantle" of the skin.
What is the function of the "acid mantle?"*
Those who study the skin's chemistry have established that its
surface normally is slightly acidic due to small quantities of
organic acids found among the secretions of the skin surface,
and to the acidic content of moisture (containing dissolved
carbon dioxide) dissolved on its surface. The acidity is altered
temporarily by cleansing with soap or detergent and water.

Scientists are not sure whether this acidity has any health
significance. Neither are they aware of any threat to the main-
tenance of normal skin functions or integrity that might arise
from temporary changes in the acidity of the skin surface
within the range of mild acid to mild base. It has been shown
that the effect of alkali alone (as found in most toilet soaps)
is negligible. Also, in normal use, there is no correlation between alkalinity of soap and irritation.

22

Esthetic Surgery

SKIN PLANING FOR ACNE SCARS

Will skin planing remove pits and scars that remain after acne? How much does it cost?

Dermabrasion (skin planing) is a recommended procedure for improving the appearance of scars and pits that remain after acne. It will not remove scars, but sometimes tends to reduce their size and depth, making them less noticeable. Not all types of scars are helped, nor are all helped equally.

However, complications such as hyperpigmentation (darkened skin areas) occasionally occur. Consultation with a physician experienced and competent in this area (usually a dermatologist or plastic surgeon) is necessary to determine whether dermabrasion is likely to be helpful in a given case.

While some physicians perform dermabrasion as an office procedure, others prefer to have their patients hospitalized. The cost of the operation depends on several factors, including the size of the area to be treated. This should be discussed with the physician who performs the procedure.

Many physicians take a conservative approach to this technique. They believe that only some patients inquiring about dermabrasion have the kind of problem for which dermabrasion ought to be seriously considered, and, of those treated, not all will be satisfied with the results. The person with leathery, pitted, wide-pored skin, most anxious for and most in need of help, can be disappointed with dermabrasion.

The first dermabrasion gives the most improvement. Secondary or repeat dermabrasion gives a proportionately reduced improvement.

Following dermabrasion the patient cannot be exposed to sun (e.g. swimming, tennis, etc.) or take birth control pills for a 6-month period. Otherwise there is a risk of splotchy hyperpigmentation of the sanded area.

WHAT SKIN PLANING INVOLVES

What does dermabrasion (skin planing) involve?
In dermabrasion, the skin is frozen and a rapidly rotating brush is stroked across the face to remove the upper layers of skin.

Swelling and extensive crusting develop in the first 24 to 48 hours. Then the crusts are shed spontaneously in 10 to 14 days, leaving the skin underneath thinner and therefore more pink than before. The skin approaches normal within 6 weeks to 6 months in most cases. The color discrepancy is masked by makeup.

Only a physician trained in the techniques of this operation should perform it because the operation is by no means a simple or rapid procedure. It requires skill and extensive training so that the danger of unsightly scarring is minimized.

SUPERFICIAL CHEMOSURGERY FOR WRINKLES

Does superficial chemosurgery (skin peeling) effectively remove wrinkles? Is this procedure safe?
Chemical peel is a procedure that destroys living tissue by the action of such caustic chemical agents as phenol or trichloroacetic acid. While physicians have used chemical cauterants mainly to treat small, benign lesions and chronic inflammatory patches for more than a hundred years, extensions and modifications of chemical peel have recently been used for the esthe-

tic improvement of sun-damaged, aged, and wrinkled skin. In this procedure, referred to as superficial chemosurgery, caustic agents are used to destroy rather extensive areas of the epidermis (outer layer of the skin) and the uppermost dermis (inner layer of the skin). It is a controlled second-degree chemical burn.

This treatment is very effective in the improvement of perioral (around the mouth) and periorbital (around the eyes) wrinkling. No other modality has given as satisfactory a result.

The American Medical Association's Committee on Cutaneous Health and Cosmetics condemns the use of superficial chemosurgery by nonmedical personnel. The dangers inherent in this practice are compounded by the use of agents for which the chemical composition is not divulged.

Since the aging process continues, the results will fade with time proportionate to the patient's aging tendency.

FACELIFT FOR WRINKLES

Will facelifting correct wrinkles? How long does it last?
The facelifting operation is carried out to ameliorate redundancy and sagging of the face and neck that appear as a person grows older. The patient should have thorough understanding of the type of operation contemplated, the possible complications and the healing time. Not all people are acceptable for plastic surgery. A careful analysis of the person, the "defect," and the indicated correction is necessary in each case.

Redundancy resulting from gravity and loss of elasticity in the skin will be markedly improved by a facelifting operation. Wrinkles formed by excessive use of the muscles of expression about the eyes and mouth, forehead and brows, may be temporarily improved by a facelifting operation, but most of these wrinkles will quite naturally persist or promptly reappear.

If the technique is successful, the patient should have the appearance he or she had 5 to 10 years earlier. However, no operation will keep anyone eternally youthful. The patient will always appear younger and the facelift effect is permanent, but aging will occur from the day of the operation forward at the normal aging process rate for that individual.

CARE FOLLOWING FACELIFTING

I recently had a surgical facelift and would like to know what general precautions I should follow to maintain the improved appearance achieved by the operation. Are particular types of creams or facial exercises available that are either helpful or harmful?

Anyone who has a facelift (or other type of plastic or dermatologic surgery such as dermabrasion or superficial chemosurgery) should obtain instructions about care from the physician who performs the operation. Specific questions should be directed to the physician during the recovery period, and afterward as needed.

Some general instructions for care following facelifts may be applicable. After the facelifting operation has been accomplished and the skin has been stretched and repositioned, the patient should try to break any personal habits that may contribute to the formation of wrinkles. For instance, some authorities say that excessive smiling (is there such a thing?) should be minimized, since they believe it helps form fine lines and wrinkles around the eyes and mouth.

Keeping a regular weight level is also helpful. Skin becomes less elastic with age, so skin stretched due to overweight may remain overstretched following weight loss, contributing to folds and sagging skin.

Unfortunately, no single muscle exercise and no single emollient or face cream will overcome the basic physiologic conditions relating to the skin and tissues of the face and neck. Emollient creams will help to "soften" aging skin temporarily, reduce dryness and roughness, and make fine lines less noticeable as long as they are used regularly. But as soon as use is discontinued the skin reverts to its "normal" state.

Some facelifts appear to last longer than others, depending on the inherent tendency either to age or to appear youthful. Therefore it is imperative for the patient to be realistic and to accept the fact that aging is inevitable.

MINI-FACELIFTS

I have read about a "15-minute facelift," developed by a French plastic surgeon, that can be performed in the doctor's office and costs much less than a regular facelift. How successful is the operation? Is it available in the United States?

The so-called "mini-facelift" is not a new technique. It is a minor surgical procedure that can be performed in the surgeon's office under local anesthesia.

A triangle of skin is cut out of the area of the temple above the hairline. The edges of skin are then sewn together, "lifting" the lower part of the face.

This procedure provides little or no improvement in the middle or upper third of the face. The degree of improvement provided to the lower third is slight and the results are quickly lost. The effects are usually not too gratifying either to the patient or to the surgeon.

PLASTIC SURGERY ON THE NOSE

I would appreciate some information on rhinoplasty. Is it very expensive? Does it require hospitalization?

The rhinoplasty operation, carried out to improve the appearance of the nose, is now a well-accepted operative technique. The operation is usually performed under local anesthesia and requires a short hospitalization. Both plastic surgeons and otolaryngologists perform this operation. After one to two weeks all bandages are off the nose, most of the swelling has disappeared, and the patient is ready to resume normal activity.

The rhinoplasty operation is not as expensive as some

other types of surgery. Costs vary depending on several factors. Discuss costs and specific questions with the surgeon you consult.

This operation is not indicated for children under age sixteen because the nose has not yet finished its natural growth or attained its adult form.

In some people the nasal septum in the nasal cavity is deviated, causing some obstruction to breathing. The operation to correct this is called a submucous resection and is often combined with the rhinoplasty technique.

PLASTIC SURGERY TO INCREASE BREAST SIZE

I would appreciate some information on plastic surgery to enlarge the size of my breasts. Are silicone gel implants preferred to other materials implanted surgically to increase breast size?

In the past 20 years significant improvements have been made in augmentation mammaplasty (plastic surgical techniques for breast enlargement). This is due mainly to the development of implants of synthetic materials. Earlier methods that entailed transplanting some of the patient's own tissue were not satisfactory.

The purpose of the implant (prosthesis) is to provide a certain amount of bulk behind the breast tissue, thus pushing the breast outward. The prosthesis is never placed within the breast tissue. The degree of breast enlargement will depend on the amount of tissue available in the general body conformation. The woman contemplating augmentation mammaplasty should let the surgeon she consults choose the material to be implanted.

Silicone gel and inflatable silastic rubber implants are among the preferred synthetic materials presently used for augmentation mammaplasty. They consist of a thin envelope or bag made of silastic (silicone rubber) and filled with silicone in gel form, dextron or saline. These implants should not be confused with the controversial, illegal technique involving injections of free liquid silicone. The latter technique is uniformly condemned by all authorities and can produce blindness and even death. (See Q and A on silicone injections later in this chapter.)

APPEARANCE OF BREASTS AFTER AUGMENTATION SURGERY

How natural do breasts look after augmentation mammaplasty?

The ideal breast prosthesis should have a delicate framework, resilient enough to hold its basic form, yet sensitive to applied pressure. Although the hard prostheses used in the past have been modified in materials and design, the ideal breast implant has not yet been developed.

Implanted breasts feel firmer than normal breasts, but the more fat and breast tissue overlying the implant, the softer and more natural the breast feels. If the patient does not have sufficient breast tissue over the prosthesis, the breasts feel quite hard and, although the contour may be pleasing to the patient, the firmness may be a source of annoyance.

To date there is no such thing as a natural-feel prosthesis. In thin patients the breasts are globe-like in appearance and may show implant folds and wrinkling through the skin. However, most patients are very gratified by the protrusion accomplished.

COMPLICATIONS FROM BREAST AUGMENTATION SURGERY

Will there be complications or permanent scars following breast augmentation surgery?

All surgical procedures including breast enlargement have certain inherent risks and a certain incidence of complications. There will be permanent scars about the breasts, although usually they are not large and conspicuous, and there will be varying degrees of discomfort and pain during the 2 to 4 weeks following surgery.

BREAST AUGMENTATION SURGERY AND CANCER

Will augmentation mammaplasty cause cancer of the breast?

Exhaustive studies with the currently available inert materials have shown that they are harmless to the patient. Although use of these prostheses does not cause cancer, we cannot assume that cancer will not develop. The incidence of breast cancer among women who have had augmentation mammaplasty will be the same as among women who have not. Any woman who cannot accept this premise is not a good candidate for surgery.

PLASTIC SURGERY FOR SAGGING BREASTS

At one time I had firm, well-shaped if rather small, breasts. Now, since I have had three children, my breasts sag and have become even smaller. What causes this condition? Can it be corrected by plastic surgery? How much would plastic surgery cost and what would it involve?

Your condition seems fairly common in women who have had one or more pregnancies. Breasts often sag and flatten following pregnancy. Physicians believe this happens mainly because the breasts' elastic tissue is repeatedly stretched and disrupted by increases in size during pregnancies. Significant weight loss that includes the breasts can also be a factor in producing this condition.

Plastic surgery can improve the condition if the patient is a suitable candidate, both physically and emotionally. A surgeon experienced in this type of plastic surgery could explain which method, if any, would be appropriate for your particular case. The surgeon would also be able to answer specific ques-

tions you may have about the operation and provide an estimate of costs.

A breast augmentation operation, insertion of a plastic
implant to raise overlying tissue, may correct the condition
satisfactorily when only a mild degree of sagging is present.
(See preceding questions in this chapter for additional information on the breast augmentation operation.)

More severely sagging breasts may require a more extensive operation, called mastopexy, in which the breasts are improved by removal of excess skin and tissue. This operation
ordinarily takes several hours. The patient is usually hospitalized for 3 to 6 days and visible permanent scars result.

Many health insurance plans do not cover esthetic surgery, so you will have to check your policy to be certain about
its provisions.

SILICONE INJECTIONS FOR BREAST ENLARGE-MENT

*How safe and effective are silicone injections for increas-
ing breast size?*

The Food and Drug Administration has prohibited distribution of medical-grade liquid silicone for the purpose of increasing breast size.

In 1965, the FDA declared that liquid silicone intended
for injections into humans for cosmetic or medical purposes
was a drug for which safety and effectiveness had not been
established. Since that time, distribution of medical-grade
liquid silicone for injections into humans has been limited to a
panel of medical specialists who have been carrying out controlled studies to determine the safety and effectiveness of the
treatment. The FDA specifically excluded the mammary
(breast) area from these controlled studies.

The possibility that injected silicone will mask malignancy
is the primary disadvantage of this method of breast augmentation. When liquid silicone is injected into tissue, numerous

globules of the plastic are formed, each one surrounded by a layer of cells. These "pseudocysts" may confuse the picture and make detection of breast malignancy by physical examination or mammography (X ray) more difficult. Small amounts of injected silicone move from the site of injection; what happens to this displaced silicone is not yet fully understood.

In contrast to silicone injections, accepted plastic surgery operations for breast augmentation do not interfere with the detection of malignancy. These operations use prostheses made of various synthetic materials, including silastic rubber bags filled with silicone gel, dextron, or saline, that are inserted under the breast tissue. As the patient's own tissue covers the mammary prosthesis entirely, any mass developing in the breast can be readily detected.

In addition, liquid silicones used by nonauthorized physicians are not the pure medical-grade products available only to registered investigators. Injection with these substitute liquids may expose the patient to further unnecessary hazards. If silicone liquid is injected past the chest wall into the lungs, silicone pneumonitis and death may result. If the liquid accidentally finds its way into a blood vessel, blindness may result.

For all of these reasons, breast augmentation by liquid silicone injections should not be performed. Women interested in breast enlargement should consult a physician experienced in plastic surgery regarding the breast augmentation operation discussed in the preceding answers.

SILICONE INJECTIONS FOR WRINKLES

Please send me the names of physicians in my area qualified to give silicone injections to remove wrinkles.

At this time, the Federal Food and Drug Administration limits the use of silicone injections for soft-tissue augmentation to a small number of registered investigators carrying out studies to determine the safety and effectiveness of the treatment. One of the unsolved problems as yet is the potential of this technique to cause late reactions (years after the injections are made).

The person with wrinkles or other problems who hopes that silicone injections will improve them should consult a physician experienced in esthetic surgery. Other treatments for these conditions do exist, and the physician can determine which, if any, is appropriate for a particular case.

The American Medical Association does not maintain lists of physicians for patient referral. You may obtain names of physicians in your area from your county medical society. Local medical societies are familiar with the abilities of physicians in their respective areas.

SAFE EAR PIERCING

I want to have my ears pierced. Is it safe to have the piercing done by a girl friend or at a jewelry store that sells earrings for pierced ears? Or should I have it done by a physician?

If you wish to have your ears pierced, you should have the operation performed by a physician. It takes only a few minutes, is relatively painless, and the possibility of infection and other complications is minimal.

Piercing performed by a friend or any unskilled person greatly increases the possibility of complications. Instruments used for piercing are not always sterile, and proper precautions often are not followed during healing. Serious internal infections, such as hepatitis, can be contracted if you have your ears pierced under unsterile conditions.

A physician first carefully measures and marks the ears because both ears may not be exactly alike. After piercing them with a sterile needle or other instrument, the physician inserts either earrings or metallic wires. Regular earrings may be inserted at this time. However, these "starter" earrings or wires should be worn for three or four weeks, until the wounds heal. They should not be removed before this time except in the case of infection or for other medical reasons. New earrings should not be inserted until the wounds are completely healed.

This is a critical period; your physician's instructions should be carefully followed to prevent infections or closure of the opening. Once the opening is established it will remain for life, unless irritation or infection results in closure.

A physician will not pierce ears that show any type of rash or infection, nor can they be pierced if multiple small sebaceous cysts are present in the ear lobes.

People subject to keloids (scar overgrowth) or who have this tendency in their families should not have their ears pierced.

SELF-EAR-PIERCERS

I have seen earrings advertised that claim to pierce ears safely and painlessly while they are being worn. Is this a safe way to pierce ears?

The small, self-piercing earring loops that are being promoted across the country are not considered safe. These devices have sharp points that are supposed to pierce ears within a few days as they are being worn. Advertisements claim that the method is inexpensive and painless, and that it will not cause infections because the self-piercers are made of 14-karat gold. Unfortunately, they do not seem to live up to their claims—infections requiring medical treatment have developed from their use. Furthermore, it is not possible to be certain that the piercers are evenly placed on the ear lobes.

If you wish to have your ears pierced, you should have the operation performed by a physician.

EARRINGS FOR PIERCED EARS

I plan to have my ears pierced and would like to know whether I have to be careful about what kind of metal is present in the earrings I wear.

People with pierced ears, especially if recently pierced, should wear earrings of known composition that do not contain nickel, a metal that causes allergic skin reactions more frequently than do other metals used for jewelry. Sterling silver does not contain nickel and rarely causes allergic reactions; neither does gold if it is 14-karat or heavier. White gold and German silver contain nickel and are known to cause reactions in nickel-sensitive persons. Costume jewelry, class rings, and the metal used for watchbands and the backs of watches often contain nickel alloys, as do metal hooks, clasps, and tabs on undergarments. Evidently some earrings for pierced ears also contain nickel. Physicians see allergic skin reactions due to nickel among patients with pierced ears who state that the earrings they wear are made of gold or silver.

Mechanical, physical, or chemical injury to the skin followed by contact with sensitizing allergens favors the development of allergic reactions. Thus, close contact with nickel-containing jewelry before the openings of pierced ears have healed can induce nickel sensitivity.

Once a person becomes allergic to nickel, the sensitivity is usually permanent and a skin reaction may develop whenever he or she comes in contact with nickel.

SURGERY FOR BAGS UNDER EYES

I am only twenty-seven years old but have developed very unattractive bags under my eyes. My physician has checked me for allergies and internal causes, but says the test results are negative. Can the condition be improved by surgery?

Plastic surgery of the eyelids to correct bags and wrinkles caused by heredity or aging is called blepharoplasty (BLEF'-ah-ro-plas'-tee). There is one operation for the upper lids and another for the lower. Each takes about an hour with hospitalization for about one day. When surgery of both upper and lower lids is needed, a combined operation is performed with the same period of hospitalization required. Swelling and discoloration generally subside within 2 weeks and scars are usually well camouflaged. The results are more lasting than those of some other types of plastic surgery (such as facelifting) because the skin on the upper part of the face stretches less with age than that on the lower part of the face.

Consult a physician experienced in plastic surgery for specific details about surgery for your problem.

The bags themselves are due to a formation of fat that normally cushions the globes of the eyes. The wrinkling results from laxity and redundancy of the lids with age. Some swelling may result from retention of body fluids and is not correctable by surgery.

EYELID SURGERY

The skin above my eyelids droops over my eyes, making them appear much smaller than they actually are. A friend of mine has suggested that I have an "eyebrow lift." What is this operation? Is it entirely safe? At age sixteen, am I old enough to undergo this surgery? Where would I find a reliable and skilled plastic surgeon?

Plastic surgery can correct some cases of hanging upper lids that do not open fully, but other cases may require different types of treatment. Drooping or hanging upper lids have various causes and the form of treatment, if any, depends on the cause.

Drooping eyelids are rare at your age unless they have been present since infancy (in which case you would have been aware of them sooner), so it is possible that you are excessively concerned about a slight variation from normal. Consult your family physician or a specialist, such as a plastic surgeon or an ophthalmologist, before you consider any type of surgery. Information on plastic surgery of the eyelids is provided in the preceding answer.

An eyebrow lift is an operation to improve sagging brows (not eyelids) and leaves in place a scar across the temple area.

CORRECTING PROTRUDING EARS

My young son is very concerned about his large, protruding ears because his classmates tease him about them constantly. Is there any way to improve the appearance of protruding ears?

Protruding, flattened, or deformed ears can be improved by plastic surgery. The operation, called otoplasty, consists of incisions behind the ears. Most frequently done in childhood, principally for social reasons, it may also be performed on adults. Both visual and psychological improvement after surgery may be dramatic.

The operation takes from 1 to 1½ hours, and the patient is usually discharged from the hospital the day after surgery. A bandage is worn over the ears for about a week, with protection during sleep for another two weeks.

This operation is not performed until the ear is almost fully grown, just prior to entering school, at about age five.

REMOVING TATTOOS

What methods are available for the removal of tattoos?

Tattoos may be removed by various surgical methods. None is completely satisfactory, however, because the pigment in a tattoo extends very deep into the skin and a scar will often result from removal by any means.

Often small tattoos can best be removed by one or more surgical excisions, leaving minimal scarring. While larger tattoos do not lend themselves as well to surgical excision, the surgical procedure can be modified to produce superficial scars. Scarification of this type, performed to obliterate pictures and names, may be sufficient to disguise the original tattoo.

Tattooing flesh-colored pigment over the original tattoo in an attempt to cover it up has not been satisfactory, since it is impossible to completely cover dark blue-black pigment with flesh-colored pigment. Furthermore, tattooed areas may contrast undesirably with tanned skin, since the tattooed areas will not tan.

Dermabrasion (skin planing) is a very poor treatment with severe limitations. It exchanges a tattoo for an unsightly scar.

For additional information on dermabrasion and a new adaptation of dermabrasion that some physicians believe is more successful, see the following answer.

NEW METHOD OF TATTOO REMOVAL

When I was in the Navy, I had a large tattoo put on my upper arm. Now I would like to have it removed. I have heard about various treatments, but none seems completely effective. Are there any new removal methods?

As you indicate, there have been few completely satisfactory methods of tattoo removal. As the preceding answer states, small tattoos often may be removed by one or more surgical excisions with minimal scarring. Most methods for removing large tattoos end in exchanging a tattoo for an obvious scar or skin discoloration.

Dermabrasion, or skin planing, is a procedure that involves removing the upper layers of skin (see answers at beginning of chapter for details of procedure). When the regular dermabrasion technique is used for tattoo removal, the physician tries to remove all skin containing tattoo pigment. Since tattoo pigment is located deep in the skin, a considerable amount of skin is removed. This can heal only with scar formation. In addition, the area will usually remain hairless and possess a different color from that of surrounding skin.

A recent adaptation of dermabrasion for tattoo removal

is superficial dermabrasion, a procedure in which the skin over the tattooed area is lightly dermabraded until it becomes irritated. The physicians who developed this technique believe it leads to an inflammatory reaction that causes certain cells to pick up the tattoo pigment and work their way to the skin surface. In some cases, one treatment has been sufficient to remove the tattoo pigment. If one treatment is not enough, the remaining pigment frequently can be removed by repeating the superficial dermabrasion after an appropriate interval.

Although superficial dermabrasion has been successful in some degree, a completely satisfactory method of tattoo removal has yet to be developed. The person who has a tattoo removed will almost always be left with scarring or another defect. Thus he must decide which is preferable—the tattoo or the defect that remains after treatment.

TATTOOS AND TABLE SALT

Is it true that doctors can now use ordinary table salt to remove tattoos?

The procedure is called salabrasion and, although it makes use of table salt, it shouldn't be attempted at home because of the danger of possible infection. In this procedure, a physician rubs table salt over the tattooed area until the skin becomes irritated.

As with superficial dermabrasion, the irritation produced by salabrasion apparently sets up an inflammatory reaction within the skin, causing certain cells to pick up the tattoo pigment and work their way to the surface. One treatment usually is sufficient, but it may be a few days before the tattoo fades.

Tattoos can also be cut out or faded through other processes, but there's always the danger of damaging the skin. It might remain hairless or have a different color from that of the surrounding skin.

The choice of treatment and the final results depend on size and location of the tattoo and other factors. This choice should be left to a physician.

LASER THERAPY FOR BIRTHMARKS AND TATTOOS

What is laser therapy and what is its status as a treatment for removing tattoos and birthmarks?

Laser therapy uses a form of intense light. There is no one laser; there are red, blue-green, and even colorless lasers. A laser may be pulsed—that is, the beam may come at intervals and may last for 1/1,000,000 of a second—or it may be continuous.

Because tattoos and birthmarks are colored and color absorbs light, the laser has been used in investigating treatments of these conditions, but not as a conventional treatment. The laser has been used only for those tattoos that cannot be treated by various types of surgery, and researchers indicate that it will remain an investigative treatment for some time.

The ruby laser is used for the treatment of tattoos, pulsed from a few thousandths of a second to a few billionths of a second. The tattoo is burned and crusts, after which it heals. Scarring and infection are possible, and if the tattoo is very large a longer term of treatment will be necessary.

In the usual method of treatment, a few areas are treated, then watched by the physician and patient for several months. If these preliminary treatments have removed the tattoo color effectively and if skin scarring is not excessive, more treatments are given. Results of the investigative studies over the years have been good.

The birthmark most often considered for investigative laser treatment is port-wine stain because its treatment by other means is generally not acceptable. Special masking cosmetics, theatrical makeup, electrodesiccation and occasionally tattooing are the currently available methods of minimizing the disfigurement of this persistent birthmark. Often plastic surgery is not possible if these permanent birthmarks cover a large area.

Test trials of laser therapy for birthmarks usually are done at age six or seven, when a child is able to cooperate. Small areas are treated as a trial and are watched by the physician and the family for several months before more extensive treatments are used. Some patients respond very well with considerable persistent lightening; others do not show any response. The darker the port-wine stain, the more effective the laser treatment. Scarring, if it develops, usually is minimal and may become less noticeable as time goes by.

It is important to emphasize that these are investigative treatments, even though they have been done for several years. At present, laser treatments of tattoos and birthmarks are conducted only in a few research centers. Specially designed laboratories and planned safety programs are required, and patients must be referred by a physician.

REMOVING "BEAUTY MARKS"

I want to have a couple of ugly moles removed from my face. How is this done?
Several methods are available. Most can be performed quickly in a physician's office. Let your physician decide which method of removal is best for your particular case. Size, location, and other factors will influence the decision.

Generally, a mole is completely removed and a scar is left in its place.

Usually a mole will not return once it has been completely removed. If it does begin to reappear, consult your physician.